DOWN WITH HIGH
BLOOD
PRESSURE

DOWN WITH HIGH BLOOD PRESSURE

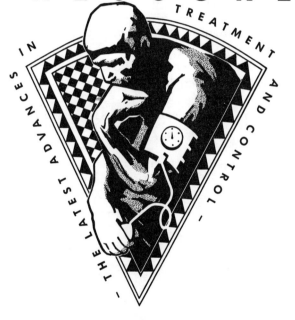

– THE LATEST ADVANCES IN TREATMENT AND CONTROL –

GROSVENOR HOUSE

The Publisher wishes to express its gratitude to **Astra Pharma Inc.** for an education grant which has helped to make the publication of this book possible.

Canadian Cataloguing in Publication Data

Haynes, R. Brian (Robert Brian), 1943 -
 Down with High Blood Pressure

Issued also in French under title: À bas l'hypertension!

ISBN 0-919959-51-2
1. Hypertension. I. Leenen, Frans H.H. II. Title.

RC685.H8H39 1990 616.1'32   C90-090196-9

Published by:

Grosvenor House Press Inc.	Éditions Grosvenor inc.
111 Queen Street East	1456, rue Sherbrooke ouest
Suite 456	3ᵉ étage
Toronto, Ontario M5C 1S2	Montréal, Québec H3G 1K4

The opinions expressed in this book are those of the authors. Readers are advised to consult with a physician prior to acting on the basis of material contained herein. The authors and Grosvenor House Press Inc. hereby disclaim any responsibility for any loss suffered by any person which results from a failure to so consult with a physician.

Table of Contents

Introduction

On behalf of the Canadian Hypertension Society, we are proud to present a new book for people who have high blood pressure (hypertension) or who want to know about this common problem. The Society's first book on this subject was published in 1986 as part of our public education program. The public's response was enthusiastic, and it convinced us that people with high blood pressure do want information about their condition. It also led us to believe that our approach to providing information was useful.

We learned from readers' letters that the information in the first book was incomplete. Our readers were particularly interested in more details about the treatments their doctors had prescribed for them. That has been one of the main reasons for this new book, and we've increased the amount of information about both drug and non-drug treatments.

Another reason for the new book is the tremendous growth in knowledge over the last four years about high blood pressure and its management. Because so many people have high blood pressure and because hypertension is one of the few chronic diseases that can be treated successfully, though not perfectly, research in this field is intense. Members of the Canadian Hypertension Society have made important contributions to this research. In addition, the Society has taken a leadership role in keeping on top of advances in the hypertension field around the world. During the last four years, the Society has held national consensus conferences on several important topics, including hypertension and diabetes mellitus, hypertension and the elderly, and treatment with and without drugs. The resulting experts' recommendations are explained in this book.

HYPERTENSION FROM THE PERSPECTIVE OF TODAY'S PATIENTS

Of all the many advances in health care over the last three decades, one of the most remarkable is the development of effective treatments for high blood pressure. Before these treatments became available, people who had hypertension were at great risk of strokes, heart failure, heart attacks, and kidney failure. Now, with good care, most of these complications can be avoided.

It should be stated that the treatments for high blood pressure aren't perfect. First, they don't cure the condition; rather, they bring blood pressure down to normal levels, and only when taken regularly. Second, the medications can cause adverse effects. Some people find taking medical treatments on a daily basis an unbearable nuisance. Some refuse entirely to take pills, and try to get by with non-drug treatments such as weight reduction, low-salt diets, giving up alcohol, and "taking it easy." Alas, these treatments are less effective than medications — and can be at least as much nuisance. But they can often complement drug treatments and reduce the need for medication.

Fortunately, there are many treatment options for high blood pressure. By matching the treatments to the individual's characteristics and responses, it's usually possible to find a successful match: good blood pressure control with few or no adverse effects.

Achieving the best match takes teamwork, however. If you have high blood pressure, the members of the team are you and your doctor, and often members of your family. Nurses, pharmacists and dietitians may also become members of your team. Your doctor's job is to know about causes and management of high blood pressure, and to know enough about you to prescribe the treatment that best fits your circumstances. Your tasks are to know enough about high blood pressure to help in this process, to follow the treatment as prescribed (or to tell your doctor if you're unable to follow it), and to report any adverse effects that you feel the treatment may be causing. Your doctor may give you additional tasks such as measuring your own blood pressure.

This book provides the facts you'll need to understand the nature of high blood pressure, its (potential) complications, and the details of its diagnosis, treatments and monitoring. This information will help you to keep up your end of the teamwork (or *therapeutic alliance*) that's needed to keep your blood pressure under control with a minimum of side-effects and fuss.

ABOUT THE AUTHORS

The authors of the book are all members of the Canadian Hypertension Society, an organization dedicated to research and education about high blood pressure. Most of us are health professionals: doctors, nurses, dietitians. Most are also involved in research on hypertension. All of us teach students in the health sciences about hypertension, and we all try to teach our patients about high blood pressure. That's why we've written this book.

ABOUT THE BOOK

This book provides an overview of hypertension. Some readers may want to read the whole book, others may want to read only the chapters of special interest to them. For those who want to select specific chapters, the following guide may help.

The first chapter describes the nature of high blood pressure and its effects on the body. If you don't know anything about blood pressure or what hypertension is, this is the place to start. However, the chapter doesn't have much practical information about what you can do to help with the treatment of your high blood pressure.

Chapter 2 provides a practical guide on how blood pressure is measured and how hypertension is diagnosed. It then explains the questions doctors ask and the tests they recommend when they see someone with newly discovered hypertension.

Chapter 3 summarizes the evidence that treatment for high blood pressure does more good than harm. If you have any doubts that blood pressure lowering treatments are beneficial, be sure to read this chapter. We think you'll be convinced!

Chapter 4 is about diet and hypertension. Diet is an aspect of lifestyle, of course, but it's so important to health that we've given it its own chapter.

Chapter 5 summarizes the relationship between lifestyle (stress, exercise, smoking, alcohol) and high blood pressure. It then provides a practical guide on how you can modify your lifestyle to lower your blood pressure.

Chapter 6 describes the current Canadian Hypertension Society recommendations on medications for high blood pressure. It's a summary of the same information given to doctors.

Chapters 7–11 provide specific details about the many medications that lower blood pressure. Here you'll find out about the effectiveness of the medications and their individual advantages and disadvantages, including side-effects.

Chapters 12–14 provide special information for specific groups: chapter 12 is for the elderly, chapter 13 for diabetics, and chapter 14 for women who are pregnant or on birth control pills.

Chapter 15 gives practical tips on what you can do to benefit most from treatment for your hypertension. This chapter is a "must" for everyone on therapy for high blood pressure.

ABOUT THE SPONSOR FOR THE BOOK

This book has been prepared with the assistance of an educational grant from Astra Pharma Inc., a pharmaceutical company that makes a variety of drugs, including some that are useful for the treatment of hypertension. We're grateful for Astra's aid, which was of particular help in publicizing the book and making it available to doctors for their patients.

We're also grateful for Astra's agreement to, and insistence on, the writing arrangements for the book. The material in this book is entirely the responsibility of the authors, on behalf of the Canadian Hypertension Society. We have attempted to represent all aspects of hypertension impartially, according to scientific merit, including all drug and non-drug treatments.

R. Brian Haynes   Frans H. H. Leenen
M.D., Ph.D.   M.D., Ph.D.

1

High Blood Pressure and the Human Body

Mitchell Levine, M.D., M.Sc. and George Fodor, M.D., Ph.D.

WHAT IS BLOOD PRESSURE ?

As the term indicates, blood pressure is the pressure by which the blood is circulated in blood vessels. The heart is a muscular pump that supplies the pressure to move the blood along. Blood vessels have elastic walls and provide some resistance to the flow. Hence, there is pressure in the system even between heart beats.

In 1733, an English clergyman and scientist named Stephen Hales made the first direct measurement of blood pressure in an animal. Hales was astonished when, upon inserting a long glass tube into an artery in the neck of a horse, the blood in the column rose 275 centimetres (nine feet).

Blood pressure varies from animal to animal. It's very high in the giraffe, where the blood must travel a long way up the neck to get to the head. In many species, including small laboratory animals, blood pressure is similar to that in humans.

11

Nature's purpose in keeping blood pressure at a certain level is to ensure that the blood, which carries nutrients and oxygen, is pumped to various organs. From the larger arteries at the heart, blood travels to smaller ones until it reaches tiny vessels, called capillaries, found in every organ and muscle. In these tiny capillaries, oxygen and energy-containing substances such as glucose cross through the vessel walls to the organs, providing them with all that's needed to make them work properly. Then the darker, oxygen-depleted blood returns through the veins to the lungs to pick up more oxygen, after which it goes back to the heart.

Blood pressure is highest in the larger arteries and lower in the smaller blood vessels. It also varies throughout the day, increasing during exercise, mental stress and sexual intercourse, and decreasing when the body is resting during sleep.

The first measurements of blood pressure in humans were taken by inserting a tube into an artery — an inconvenient, somewhat dangerous, and painful method. General use of blood pressure readings was made possible by the development of so-called indirect techniques, particularly an inflatable cuff like the tube in a tire.

Blood pressure is usually indicated as two numbers; for example, 130/80 (which is expressed as "130 over 80"). The first number is the systolic pressure and the second number is the diastolic pressure, expressed in millimetres of mercury (mm Hg).

Systolic blood pressure is caused by the heart's contraction, pushing blood from the heart into the body's largest vessel, the aorta. The diastolic blood pressure occurs between contractions of the heart, when the heart itself is being filled with the blood coming from the veins and lungs. This pressure is due to the resistance in the smallest arteries, the capillaries.

If we were to repeat Stephen Hales's experiment with a glass tube filled with mercury, the pressure in the artery would raise the column of mercury 130 millimetres during the contraction of the heart. Mercury is a very heavy liquid; if we used water instead of mercury, the water would rise 256 centimetres — more than eight feet! Mercury is obviously a more convenient fluid to use.

There is more information on measuring blood pressure in chapter 2 and instructions on how you can measure your own blood pressure in chapter 15.

HOW BLOOD PRESSURE IS KEPT NORMAL

To ensure sufficient nutrient and oxygen supply to all organs, it's vital for the body to keep the blood pressure within a safe margin. Many organs of the body have messenger mechanisms to make their needs known. These organs include the brain, the kidneys, the endocrine glands, the heart and the blood vessels.

The methods by which blood pressure is maintained are complicated and not completely understood. We do know quite a bit, however, and if you would like to learn more about them, read on. Otherwise you might want to skip to the next section, *High Blood Pressure.*

The brain is the body's central control, directing the various organs in response to the body's demands and needs. The centre of blood pressure control is located in the brain. Via the nerves, incoming signals from all parts of the body inform the brain of the status of blood pressure, the volume of blood, and the specialized needs of all organs. This information is processed by the brain, decisions are automatically taken, and signals are sent out via the outgoing nerves. The nerves departing from the brain end up in the organs, including the blood vessels, where they send signals that cause narrowing or widening of the vessels as required. These nerves function automatically, without our knowledge, unlike other nerves that we can control (such as those needed for physical movements of the body). They form part of the autonomic nervous system.

At the point where the nerves end and send their information to an organ, a finely regulated key/lock type of arrangement is located in the vessels. The nerves release their message in the form of substances called neurotransmitters. These neurotransmitters serve as the "key" and fit into the "lock" (called the *receptor*), and thus are able to "open the door" of the vessel.

Blood pressure can be affected at many levels — in the brain centre, on the way to and from the autonomic nervous system, during the process of sending messages to blood vessels via the key/lock mechanism. Blood pressure medications can intervene at one or more of these levels.

The kidneys are the regulators of fluids in the body, filtering out excess amounts and keeping whatever we need for survival. These organs have many special functions that help us survive as creatures who live out of the sea, as they can keep the necessary amount of salt and water in the body while getting rid of the excess. The kidneys can also cause blood pressure to increase. This can happen if one of the arteries to a kidney becomes partly blocked. To restore the blood flow it needs, the kidney makes the hormone renin, which causes the blood pressure to rise. Blood pressure will also rise if the kidneys become diseased and begin to fail, causing the fluids of the body to back up.

Hormones from several other organs can also raise blood pressure. If the thyroid gland becomes hyperactive, producing too much thyroid hormone, the blood pressure can become increased. On top of each kidney sits a small adrenal gland. It secretes several hormones that can raise blood pressure, including cortisone and adrenaline, and aldosterone, which is responsible for maintaining enough salt for the body's survival. All of these hormones are necessary for the body to function. It's only when they are excreted in excess that they cause the blood pressure to become elevated.

The heart's main purpose is to pump blood to the body's organs. Researchers throughout the world have recently become interested in another, newly discovered function: Canadian studies have shown that the heart is also an endocrine gland, secreting natriuretic hormone. This substance rids the body of excess salt and also helps keep the blood vessels properly dilated (opened up). Thus, the heart has been found to play a direct role in regulating blood pressure.

The final participants in this process of blood pressure control are the arteries. These are elastic tubes that distribute blood throughout the body to the organs. The muscles in the walls of these vessels can dilate or contract to increase the blood supply to an organ, or to shunt blood away and distribute it where it's most needed. For example, when you eat, blood flow is increased to the bowel to help with digestion. When you exercise, your body sends more blood to the muscles, while at the same time trying to maintain the proper amount of blood for the brain and other vital organs.

The functions of the kidneys, hormones and arteries are not isolated. They are directed by the brain, but they also use their own systems to inform each other of their needs. For example, the kidney's secretion of renin is influenced by the brain; however, if the blood supply to the kidney is blocked, the kidney can secrete renin without consulting the brain. The renin is then converted into the hormone angiotensin. Angiotensin causes the arteries to constrict, or narrow, so blood pressure rises. This is good for the kidney, because it forces blood past the obstruction in the artery to the kidney. Unfortunately, the blood pressure is raised in the rest of the body as well. As you will see, this is one of the causes of high blood pressure.

HIGH BLOOD PRESSURE

The regulation of blood pressure is very complicated, and it's understandable that this system can become upset in some people. Blood pressure sometimes remains high even when the body doesn't need it. This is what we call high blood pressure (or hypertension), meaning an abnormal increase of blood pressure due to the malfunction of one or more of the factors responsible for maintaining normal blood pressure.

We must clear up a common misunderstanding here. Hypertension does *not* mean that a person is "hyper" or "tense" in the sense of being nervous. High blood pressure usually has nothing to do with stress or nervous tension. The reasons for high blood pressure are discussed in detail below.

But where does high blood pressure begin and normal blood pressure end? The authorities don't always agree on the exact number at which health ends and disease starts, but most consider blood pressure to be normal below 140/90 mmHg. Above that, the increase of blood pressure leads to important increases in the risk of heart disease, stroke, kidney damage and damage to the large blood vessels of the body.

A practical definition of high blood pressure is the level at which treatment to lower blood pressure does more good than harm. Chapter 3 provides details about this level.

LOW BLOOD PRESSURE

This book is about high blood pressure, but we'll say a few words about low blood pressure. If you don't have low blood pressure, you can skip to the next section.

In general, we don't define low blood pressure by a number, as we do for high blood pressure, but rely upon the presence of symptoms to show if there's a problem. You may have heard people say that they are tired as a result of low blood pressure. Low blood pressure may indeed cause symptoms such as fatigue, but fortunately, it doesn't have as severe complications as high blood pressure. On the other hand, when your blood pressure gets too low, your brain doesn't receive enough blood and you get dizzy. If this continues, you can faint, especially when you stand up. This certainly can be a nuisance and can sometimes have serious consequences — for example, if you fall and break a bone. There are several treatments for this problem, and you should consult your doctor if you become very lightheaded upon standing up.

CAUSES OF HIGH BLOOD PRESSURE

As we mentioned a few paragraphs ago, there are many factors involved in the control of blood pressure. Upsets in any of these factors can lead to high blood pressure. However, in almost 95 percent of cases we don't know why a person's blood pressure becomes elevated; none of the factors that we can measure seems to be upset. In other words, although we know quite a bit about how the body controls blood pressure, we simply don't know much about what causes blood pressure to become elevated. When the cause can't be determined, we call it *essential* or *primary* hypertension.

In some cases — about one in twenty — we can find the cause, such as an endocrine gland secreting an excessive amount of a hormone, or a decreasing blood supply to the kidneys. In these cases, we refer to the high blood pressure as *secondary* hypertension. Some of the causes of secondary hypertension can be cured and some cannot.

Figure 1 indicates some of the major causes of hypertension. Since only one of every 20 people with hypertension has one of the secondary causes, some of them are very rare indeed. We'll discuss each of them in order.

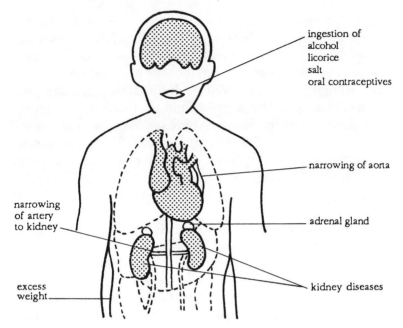

ingestion of
alcohol
licorice
salt
oral contraceptives

narrowing of aorta

narrowing
of artery
to kidney

adrenal gland

excess
weight

kidney diseases

Figure 1:   Causes of high blood pressure.

Essential hypertension

The vast majority of people with high blood pressure have essential hypertension. No doubt there are underlying causes for essential hypertension, but we don't understand them as yet. Thus medical science is still faced with an enigma about a disease that affects over ten percent of the world's adult population. On the other hand, the efforts of the last four decades have helped us to understand that, although the cause may be unknown, the basis of high blood pressure is an increase in the resistance of blood vessels to the flow of blood. Even without fully understanding some aspects of the disease, we do know how to treat it. More important, as we discuss in chapter 3, lowering blood pressure by treatment will help protect the individual from health complications.

Diseases of the kidneys

The kidneys play a very important role in the regulation of blood pressure, and it's natural that some diseases of the kidneys adversely affect blood pressure. As the function of a diseased kidney declines, blood pressure usually becomes elevated. There is often very little that can be done to cure chronic kidney disease. However, elevated blood pressure must be treated effectively to avoid further damage to the kidneys and other organs from the high blood pressure itself. This is possible with modern blood pressure-lowering medications.

Decreased blood supply to the kidneys

Hypertension caused by decreased blood supply to the kidneys is called *renovascular hypertension*. Each kidney usually receives its blood supply from a major artery called the renal artery. If this artery becomes narrowed, blood supply to the kidney may be reduced, and the kidney will then secrete renin to raise the blood pressure so the flow of blood can be restored. Unfortunately, the pressure is raised throughout the whole body system and the result is hypertension.

There are two main causes of narrowing of the arteries to the kidneys. The first and most common cause is *atherosclerosis* (hardening of the arteries), which makes the arteries narrower. This is more common in late middle age and onward. The second cause is *fibromuscular hyperplasia*. This occurs mainly in young women and may be aggravated by pregnancy. In either case, the condition can often be treated by surgery to bypass the affected artery. This procedure is a forerunner of the now famous coronary artery bypass.

More recently, a less difficult method has been developed for opening the renal artery. This is done by stretching or dilating the inside of the artery, using a catheter with a balloon at its tip. The catheter is a hollow tube, which is inserted into a major artery in the groin and is moved up into the renal artery. The tip of the catheter is placed at the site of narrowing and the balloon is then inflated through the catheter, stretching the renal artery at the narrowed section. Usually the procedure can be done in a few minutes, and the patient can go home the next day.

Primary aldosteronism

Aldosterone is a hormone secreted by the adrenal glands. It plays a role in the balance of fluid and salt in the body. If too much of the hormone is secreted — for example, by a *tumor* (abnormal tissue growth) in the adrenal gland — too much salt is retained in the body. This has the effect of raising the blood pressure. If the excess secretion of aldosterone is due to a single tumor that can be removed, surgery is usually the treatment of choice. However, if both adrenal glands are involved, the treatment is usually a medication, such as spironolactone, that blocks the effect of the aldosterone.

Coarctation of the aorta

Coarctation means *narrowing*. Narrowing of the aorta results in decreased blood supply to the lower part of the body, including the kidneys. The kidneys try to overcome this problem by secreting renin, which raises the blood pressure. Coarctation is generally a problem that a person is born with, and it causes hypertension early in life. The treatment is to surgically remove the narrowing.

Cushing's Syndrome

In this disorder, the adrenal glands secrete too much of the hormone cortisone, which can cause blood pressure to become elevated. Symptoms of Cushing's Syndrome include weight gain on the upper back and distinctive stretch marks on the abdomen. This is a complex disorder, and its management usually requires collaboration between specialists in endocrine disease and surgeons.

Oral contraceptives

Oral contraceptives that contain estrogen can raise blood pressure, sometimes to the level of hypertension. This is discussed in more detail in chapter 14. Blood pressure will often return to normal when the birth control medication is stopped. If you are taking oral contraceptives and have high blood pressure, be sure to remind your doctor.

Pheochromocytoma

This exotic-sounding problem is due to yet another disorder of the adrenal glands. The central part of the glands, called the *medulla*, secretes the hormones adrenaline and noradrenaline. A tumor can cause the medulla to become hyperactive, secreting excessive amounts of these hormones, which, in turn, can elevate the blood pressure. The excess secretion usually comes in bursts and causes characteristic symptoms including a fast, pounding heartbeat, headache, sweating and trembling. Unless you have bouts of this nature with all the symptoms at the same time, you are unlikely to have pheochromocytoma. Most of the tumors that cause pheochromocytoma are *benign* (not cancerous) and can be removed surgically. Sometimes the tumor is *malignant* (cancerous) and develops, or has spread, outside the adrenal glands by the time it's discovered and can't be treated surgically.

Other causes of hypertension

There are some other rare causes of hypertension that we won't discuss in detail here. First, excess ingestion of licorice can have an effect similar to increased aldosterone (see above) and can raise the blood pressure. The solution for this is obvious! Second, other endocrine problems such as *acromegaly* (excess secretion of growth hormone from the pituitary gland in the head) and *hyperparathyroidism* (excess secretion of hormone from the parathyroid glands in the neck) can cause elevated blood pressure. Third, hereditary diseases such as *polycystic kidney disease* cause hypertension. Fourth, it's likely that heredity determines a person's response to circumstances, such as stress or increased salt intake, that result in hypertension. These latter relationships, while not well understood, are discussed in more detail in chapters 4 and 5.

HOW HIGH BLOOD PRESSURE AFFECTS THE BODY

High blood pressure, if untreated for long periods, can cause damage to the arteries of the body and to the organs that are supplied with blood by these arteries. The major organs affected are the heart, the brain and the kidneys, as shown in figure 2.

Before going into detail, it must be emphasized that most of the complications caused by high blood pressure can be prevented if the blood pressure is brought down to normal levels by treatment. If your blood pressure is under control, you need not worry about it causing any of the problems discussed in this chapter.

It's also important to understand that factors other than hypertension can cause similar problems and that these factors should also be controlled. They include smoking, high cholesterol levels and diabetes.

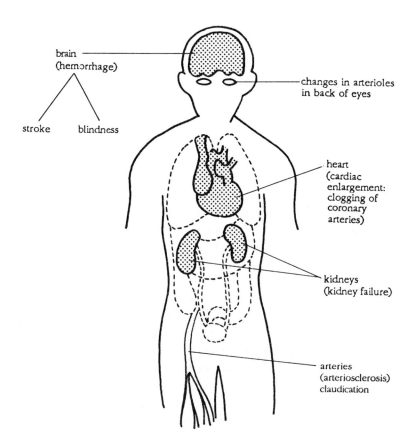

Figure 2: Target organs affected.

The heart

Like any muscle in the body forced to do extra work, the heart
becomes bigger when it has to pump against higher pressure.
Although the heart can stand high pressure for quite a long
time, eventually, over many years, it will begin to fail. When
this happens, fluid from the blood backs up into the lungs and
the lungs become "waterlogged." Because the heart has
difficulty pumping blood to the muscles when they need extra
oxygen for exercise or work, a person will feel short of breath.
At first, the shortness of breath comes on only during activity.
Eventually, breathing becomes difficult even during rest. The
technical term for this problem is *congestive heart failure.*

The heart also has its own blood supply through vessels
called the coronary arteries. The arteries to the heart can be
hardened and narrowed in the same way that arteries to other
organs are damaged. (This is discussed in detail in the next
section.) When the coronary arteries become too narrow to
carry enough oxygen for the heart to do its work, a person ex-
periences a sensation of pressure, tightness or heaviness in
the chest that lasts for about five to 15 minutes and goes away
after resting. This pain is called *angina pectoris* or *angina.* At
first, this sensation comes on only with exercise or strenuous
work. Later, it can occur with very little activity or with
excitement or emotional upset.

Although the discomfort of angina is a warning of too
little blood supply to the heart, no permanent damage is done
by it. Just lowering the blood pressure can often reduce the
work of the heart enough to relieve the angina. However, if
the blood supply to a part of the heart is blocked even more,
permanent damage is done to the heart muscle. This is called
a *heart attack,* a *coronary,* or a *myocardial infarction,* and is
usually signalled by chest pain lasting longer than that caused
by angina (typically, at least 30 minutes and often much
longer), as well as nausea and sweating. A heart attack can be

fatal but, if a person can get to the hospital in time, the chances for a good recovery are high.

The arteries

As time goes on, all humans develop hardening of the arteries (atherosclerosis) whether or not they have high blood pressure. Hardening of the arteries results in the walls of arteries becoming thicker and less elastic. This eventually begins to block blood flow. High blood pressure causes an increase in the rate at which hardening of the arteries occurs.

The arteries of the body do not all narrow at the same rate. The effects of narrowing of the arteries depend on which organs are fed by the narrowed arteries. For example, as discussed, if any artery to the heart muscle becomes blocked, the result is a heart attack. If any artery to the brain is blocked, then a stroke occurs. If the blood supply to the kidneys is blocked, then *nephrosclerosis* occurs, with the kidneys becoming shrunken and eventually failing.

The arteries to the legs can also be affected. When these arteries become narrowed, cramps in the legs, similar in nature to the cramp of the heart with angina, occur during walking. Pain due to poor blood supply to the leg muscles has the medical name of *intermittent claudication*. As with angina, this pain also goes away in a few minutes with rest. However, if the narrowing of the arteries of the legs becomes very severe, pain occurs even at rest. Eventually, the tissues of the leg, starting with the toes, die. This is called *gangrene*.

Narrowing of the arteries to the bowel also gives rise to cramps in the stomach area or just below — a condition called *abdominal angina*. Complete blockage of the blood supply to the bowel causes bleeding from the bowel and infection usually sets in, causing a person to be very sick.

If the blood pressure elevation is mild, the increase in the rate of hardening of the arteries is not great. Usually, the blood pressure must be elevated for many years before there are adverse effects. If the blood pressure is brought back to normal by treatment, the risk of complications is reduced.

If the blood pressure is severely elevated for a period of time, then the consequences come sooner and are usually much worse. Rather than gradually narrowing the vessels, severely elevated pressure can cause the blood vessels to burst. When blood leaks out of a blood vessel it is called a *hemorrhage.* Hemorrhage into the brain causes a very serious stroke that is often fatal. Severely elevated pressure can also cause the largest artery of the body, the aorta, to bulge and even burst. The bulge is called an *aneurysm,* and the bursting process is called a *dissection.* Fortunately, serious blood pressure elevations are uncommon. When they do happen, there are often warning signs before these severe problems occur. The warnings of severely elevated blood pressure include headache, nosebleeds, blurred vision, and sometimes chest pains or pains in the abdomen. Again, these complications are unlikely to occur unless high blood pressure is left untreated for a prolonged period.

The brain

Some of the effects of hypertension on the brain have already been mentioned. Blockage of an artery to a part of the brain causes a *stroke.* A person with high blood pressure has a much greater risk of stroke (about seven times the risk, on average, if the high blood pressure is untreated) than a person with normal blood pressure.

A stroke can occur in three ways. First, hardening of the arteries can lead to the inside lining of the larger arteries becoming rough and cracked. Small clots or bits of debris can collect on these roughened areas. They can then break off, becoming stuck in smaller arteries downstream. This blocks the blood supply, resulting in a stroke. The broken-off bits are called *emboli*, and this type of event is called an *embolic stroke*. Second, the narrowing in the larger arteries can be so great that the blood supply is blocked in them. This is either a direct effect of the narrowing or due to a clot forming in the narrowed artery. The result is an *atherothrombotic stroke*. Finally, if the pressure is high enough, an artery can actually burst, causing a hemorrhage into the brain — a hemorrhagic stroke. Although hemorrhagic strokes are usually the most severe, they are also the rarest. Even better, the occurrence of *hemorrhagic stroke* has been decreased more than other kinds of strokes by blood pressure lowering treatment.

We must note here that, while some strokes are very serious, many are not. In the first place, the brain has a rich blood supply, with backup routes for blood to get to most parts. As a result, complete blockage of one or even several arteries may cause no ill effects at all. Second, many people who are stroke-prone will experience warning attacks, called *transient ischemic attacks* or TIAs. These cause temporary symptoms, such as loss of vision or speech, or numbness in the hand or leg, lasting less than 24 hours and often only a few seconds. If TIAs are promptly treated, the chance of avoiding a full stroke later is 75 percent. Proper treatment usually means good control of blood pressure plus ASA (acetylsalicylic acid, or Aspirin). Who would ever have thought that this common remedy would turn out to be so useful?

The effect of a stroke depends on which area of the brain it damages. It's quite possible for a person to have several small strokes without noticing any problems at all. On the other hand, a small stroke in an important part of the brain can have devastating or even fatal effects. For example, a stroke that damages the part responsible for movement of the arm can leave someone quite crippled, particularly if that arm is the most used.

If the blood pressure is very severely elevated, then the blood vessels can break down quickly. This results in leakage of fluid and blood cells into the brain and leads to the symptoms of very severe headache and fatigue. Because the skull, in which the brain sits, does not allow any expansion, the leakage of fluid into the brain increases the pressure inside the skull and can damage the brain directly.

The good news is that over the last two decades the rate of all these complications has decreased dramatically. This is the result of the control of high blood pressure with modern treatments. High blood pressure does increase the risk of stroke, but the likelihood of your having a stroke depends on the level of blood pressure elevation. If your blood pressure is controlled, you are at no greater risk of a stroke than anyone with normal blood pressure.

The kidneys

High blood pressure can cause kidney damage, and the kidneys can also cause high blood pressure. In this section, however, we will discuss only the effects of high blood pressure on the kidney.

High blood pressure reduces the blood flow to the kidneys. This is thought to be due to an increase in the resistance in the small arteries of the kidney. Initially, the kidney's job of filtering the blood for wastes is not affected. If the hypertension continues or becomes more severe, there is eventually a greater reduction in blood flow to the kidneys. The hardening of the arteries caused by the high blood pressure adds to this problem of low blood flow.

In addition to its effect on blood flow, very high blood pressure directly damages the filtering system in the kidneys. The result is that the kidneys are no longer able to filter out wastes from the blood stream efficiently, and these consequently build up in the body. The more severe the hypertension, the more direct the damage to the filtering system.

Fortunately, kidney complications are the easiest ones to prevent. These days, we hardly ever see people with kidney failure due to hypertension.

Death

Hypertension has been called the silent killer because it usually causes very few symptoms until a considerable amount of damage has been done. The damage can then be fatal in the form of a heart attack, a stroke, or, less often, bleeding from a burst artery or kidney failure.

Because most people with hypertension have their blood pressure elevation detected before any complications occur, and because modern treatments for high blood pressure can bring the blood pressure back to normal, the term "silent killer" is rapidly becoming outdated.

Unfortunately, there are some people whose blood pressure elevation goes undetected because they seldom see a doctor. There are also patients who drop out of treatment or fail to take the treatment that has been prescribed for them. This is a tragic situation, as elevated blood pressure can be a cause of early death. It has been estimated that untreated moderate hypertension (a diastolic pressure between 105 and 120) reduces one's lifespan by an average of more than 16 years. If life indeed begins at 40, hypertension can cut short the best part of your life. If you have high blood pressure, make sure you get good treatment for it! Ways to do this are discussed in the rest of this book, particularly in chapter 15.

2

Diagnostic Tests

Richard A. Reeves, M.D. and Martin J. Bass, M.D., M.Sc.

We have four aims in this chapter: to describe how blood pressure is measured; to explain how blood pressure measurements are used to make the diagnosis of hypertension; to look at questions that doctors may ask and tests they may recommend if it's found that you do have high blood pressure; and, finally, to answer some common questions that patients with hypertension ask.

HOW BLOOD PRESSURE IS MEASURED

Measuring blood pressure is simple, quick and virtually painless. A cuff around the upper arm is filled with enough air to squeeze the artery. This temporarily stops the flow of blood. As the air in the cuff is slowly released, the doctor or nurse — or you — listens with a stethoscope as blood starts to rush through the artery. The first tapping sound that's heard is the systolic blood pressure. This is the maximum pressure produced when the heart beats. The reading is recorded as the height of the mercury column when the blood starts to flow. This is expressed as millimetres of mercury, or, in symbols, "mmHg". Systolic blood pressure usually ranges from 100 to 200 mmHg. If the systolic blood pressure is over 140 mmHg, it is considered elevated.

The measure commonly used for decisions about treatment is the diastolic blood pressure. As the air is released from the cuff, a point is reached where the artery is fully open. At this point, the blood flows smoothly and the sound over the artery disappears. The pressure when this last sound disappears is recorded as the diastolic blood pressure. This is the pressure in the arteries when the heart is between beats. Diastolic blood pressure usually ranges from 60 to 100 mmHg. Diastolic pressure below 90 mmHg is considered normal. A diastolic pressure between 90 and 104 mmHg is considered mildly elevated; between 105 and 114, moderately elevated; and over 114 mmHg, severely elevated.

For convenience, these two readings are written together. For example, "130/80" means a blood pressure of 130 mmHg systolic and 80 mmHg diastolic, and it's expressed as "130 over 80."

Blood pressures taken when you're lying, sitting or standing are usually very similar. However, some people, particularly the elderly and diabetics, may have much lower pressures when they stand up. Some drugs lower standing blood pressure more than lying blood pressure. In these situations, the pressure is often measured both while lying and standing. For treatment decisions, many doctors feel that the blood pressure taken while sitting quietly, not talking, is the best single pressure to measure, because it represents the usual way most of us spend our daytime hours.

No matter which position you're in, you must be comfortable and have your arm supported. If your arm is unsupported, the muscles have to work, and this may raise the blood pressure readings. The doctor or nurse can support your arm, or you can rest your arm on a table or the arm of a chair.

THE ROLE OF HOME BLOOD PRESSURES

Sometimes people have lower blood pressures at home than at the doctor's office. Some people also find it helpful to see the effect of their medications on their blood pressure. In addition, many doctors find it easier to adjust medications and to help people follow their treatments if blood pressures are taken between visits as well as at the clinic. These are all good reasons for purchasing a blood pressure kit so you can take your own pressure at home. If you are interested in this, see chapter 15.

All people doing self-monitoring should have a doctor or nurse whom they can contact if they're concerned. In some patients, self-monitoring of blood pressure may result in excess concern about the usual peaks of blood pressure, and in a few it may increase anxieties about health. Blood pressure varies from time to time in each of us. For example, your blood pressure could be 150/90 at one time and 120/80 just a few minutes later. This is normal. The level of blood pressure used to decide about treatment is based on the average of several readings, not on a single reading.

You may be able to obtain additional readings that will help your doctor in decisions about your treatment. If a nurse visits your home regularly, or if you can see a nurse at your workplace, have your blood pressure checked; ask the nurse to write down the readings with the date and time so you can show them to your doctor.

However, we don't recommend using machines available in public places such as shopping centres and airports. They're often quite inaccurate.

AMBULATORY BLOOD PRESSURE MONITORING

There's one more way in which your doctor may obtain information on your blood pressure. Portable automatic blood pressure measuring devices have recently become available through some doctors' offices. These devices can record blood pressures many times during the day. You wear a blood pressure cuff around your arm as you go about your usual activities, and the cuff inflates and deflates automatically under the control of a small pump contained in the equipment.

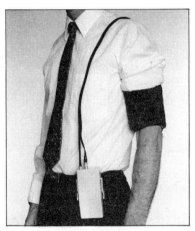

Figure 1: A light-weight ambulatory blood pressure monitor.

These machines are no bigger than a large paperback book and are worn on a belt or shoulder strap. They're reasonably comfortable to wear, and don't usually disrupt the daily routine or sleep. Information is stored in the unit's memory and later transferred to a computer to print out the results. With these machines, an average blood pressure can be determined during many different activities. The results may allow the diagnosis of hypertension to be made more accurately.

Ambulatory blood pressure monitoring isn't for everyone. It's most useful for patients who have only borderline pressure elevation, or who are suspected of having *white coat syndrome.* This is a condition in which pressure is elevated in the doctor's office but is lower away from the office. It may be suspected if measurements by family members or home pressure measurements are much lower than those found in the doctor's office, or if, despite very high pressures measured in the office, the doctor's examination reveals no evidence of damage to the body from high blood pressure.

At present, it's known that heart enlargement and other effects of high blood pressure on the body seem to depend more on home or ambulatory blood pressure than on the office blood pressure. In addition, people with white coat syndrome may be less likely to develop ill effects from high blood pressure than patients who have high pressure both in and outside the doctor's office. However, only further research will clarify whether a patient with hypertension in the office but a normal ambulatory blood pressure can safely go without treatment. For now, ambulatory blood pressure is best viewed as one more piece of information in deciding whether an elevated office blood pressure requires treatment or not.

HOW HYPERTENSION IS DIAGNOSED

Does one elevated blood pressure reading mean that you have hypertension? No! As we mentioned, blood pressure varies in all of us. There are many reasons for pressures to be high at any one time. Pressures taken just after exercise, or when you're upset or excited, may be higher as a temporary response to the situation. A blood pressure that remains high after you've sat quietly for five minutes is more important. Even then, just the situation of having one's blood pressure taken can elevate the reading. To overcome this, your doctor may measure your blood pressure twice or more during a visit and record only the lowest pressure.

Medical authorities agree that a minimum of two elevated blood pressure readings taken on at least two different days is needed to make the diagnosis of high blood pressure, or hypertension. Furthermore, research shows that blood pressures taken monthly in the doctor's office may continue to drop for up to six months. Because of this, the Canadian Hypertension Society recommends, for patients whose diastolic blood pressure appears mildly elevated, that the diagnosis of hypertension should be based on at least three blood pressure measurements over a period of six months. This period may be shortened if the blood pressure is moderately elevated or if there's any evidence of damage from the high blood pressure.

Unfortunately, there are many people who feel that they have hypertension because they once had an elevated blood pressure, even though readings after that time have usually been normal. In fact, a recent survey showed that more people with normal readings thought they had hypertension than there were people who actually had high blood pressure. If you're not on antihypertensive medication and your blood pressure is usually normal (less than 140/90 mmHg), then you do *not* have hypertension!

WHEN SYSTOLIC BLOOD PRESSURE IS IMPORTANT

Sometimes a person can have a systolic blood pressure that is high (over 140 mmHg) while the diastolic blood pressure is normal (under 90 mmHg). Because the value of treating such isolated elevations of systolic pressure remains unclear, most doctors pay closer attention to the levels of diastolic blood pressure. But elevated systolic pressure is important. If the systolic blood pressure is repeatedly above 160 mmHg while the diastolic blood pressure is below 90 mmHg, a person is considered to have *isolated systolic hypertension.*

THE DOCTOR'S INVESTIGATION OF HIGH BLOOD PRESSURE

Once the doctor is certain that you really have high blood pressure, he'll investigate further. This involves four steps (detailed in the tables at the end of this chapter): an interview about your medical history, current health and related activities (Table 1); a physical examination (Table 2); routine tests (Table 3); other tests that may be done (Table 4).

Each step may provide the answer to at least one of the following three questions: What is the *cause* of the high blood pressure? Has the high blood pressure had any lasting *effect* on your body? Are there any *other factors* that may increase your chance of having a stroke, heart problems or other complications of high blood pressure?

Finding a cause for the high blood pressure may allow partial or complete cure. If the elevated blood pressure has affected your body or you have other factors that increase the risk of a complication, it may be important to start treatment at lower levels of elevated diastolic blood pressure. We'll look into each of these three questions in the sections that follow.

WHAT IS THE CAUSE OF YOUR HIGH BLOOD PRESSURE ?

In about 95 out of 100 cases, no clear cause of high blood pressure can be found even after a thorough investigation. As explained in chapter 1, this is called primary or essential hypertension. In only about one or two out of a hundred cases is a treatable cause found. Most of the time, when a cause can be found, it cannot be cured, but the blood pressure can almost always be controlled.

The most easily treated causes of elevated blood pressure can all be discovered by simple questions or examinations. Here are some of the questions that your doctor may ask:

Are you taking any medications?

Some drugs, both prescription and non-prescription, increase blood pressure. When they're stopped, the blood pressure often returns to normal. The most commonly used drugs that can elevate blood pressure are birth control pills and pills for the menopause, both of which contain the hormone estrogen. Long-term use of cold or sinus remedies or allergy tablets can occasionally raise blood pressure. They contain decongestants that constrict the blood vessels of the nose and body. A similar effect is seen with some diet pills and herbal remedies.

What's your licorice, alcohol and salt intake? your weight?

Things that you eat and drink can affect your blood pressure. The rare person who eats a lot of licorice every day risks elevated blood pressure. The more alcohol you drink (above two drinks per day), the higher the blood pressure. This rise in pressure is quickly reversed by cutting back on alcohol. Some people's blood pressure is salt sensitive. Reduction of excessive salt intake may decrease blood pressure (see chapter 4). High blood pressure is also related to overweight. If you're one of the fortunate obese people who can lose weight, then you may well lose your high blood pressure too.

Have you been under stress recently?

A stressful situation such as a problem at work, a financial crisis or marital difficulties can raise your blood pressure temporarily. There's no good evidence that long-term stress raises blood pressure by itself. If the doctor finds that you're under stress, he may choose to have you come back at a less stressful time to recheck your blood pressure. Reduction of stress may result in a lower blood pressure.

We must note here that many people think that high blood pressure is a stress-related disease and that a person who's tense and anxious or under stress has high blood pressure. This is seldom the case. People who are stressed may have high blood pressure, but this is not often due to the stress itself. People who are relaxed and "laid back" can also have high blood pressure. The only way to tell is to have the blood pressure checked.

Have you had any problems with your kidneys?

As explained in chapter 1, the kidneys play an important role in controlling your blood pressure. Kidney problems may lead to high blood pressure. Here are some problems your doctor will look for:

Chronic renal (kidney) disease. Chronic kidney disease is the most frequent of the rare causes of high blood pressure. The doctor will search for this cause by asking questions about chronic kidney and urinary infections and pain in the region of the kidney. This can be either flank pain (between the ribs and the pelvis) or abdominal pain. Kidney injury from accidents or kidney stones is also important.

The doctor will examine your urine for protein and cells that should not be there, and will also take blood samples to test for creatinine or urea. Creatinine and urea are compounds produced by the body as it turns food into energy and forms new cells. Both are normal components of blood, and unusual levels of either can provide a clue as to how well the kidneys are functioning.

Narrowing of the artery to the kidney (renal artery stenosis). If the blood supply to one kidney is reduced because of a partial blockage, the kidney will respond by increasing the blood pressure. In some cases, the blood flowing through the narrowed artery makes a noise that can be heard through a stethoscope.

If the doctor hears this noise when listening over your abdomen, he may then order a renal scan. This test involves having a small — and safe — amount of radioactive dye injected, and then lying beneath a scanner that detects the rate at which the dye is taken up by the kidneys. Another test that is occasionally done is an *intravenous pyelogram* or IVP. This involves the injection of a small amount of liquid, called dye or contrast, that shows up on an X-ray as soon as the dye reaches the kidneys.

If a blocked artery to the kidney is still suspected after the initial tests, then an X-ray movie can be taken of the artery to the kidney. This X-ray is called an *arteriogram* or *angiogram*. A small tube is inserted through an artery in the groin and is moved inside the artery until it is near the kidney. X-ray dye is then injected. As the dye flows along the artery to the kidney, an X-ray movie will reveal any blockage or narrowing.

As final proof that a kidney with a narrowed artery is causing the high blood pressure, a *renal vein renin test* may be performed. Renin is a chemical produced by the kidney that raises blood pressure. If one kidney is causing the high blood pressure, it will be over-producing renin. This is measured through a small tube inserted into a vein in the groin and advanced up to the vein leaving each kidney.

Do you have coarctation of the aorta?

This is a narrowing of the main blood vessel coming from the heart. The narrowing reduces the flow of blood to the legs but not the arms. Therefore, the clue the doctor looks for is a delay between the pulse in your wrist and in your groin, or a higher blood pressure in your arm than in your leg.

Do you have any problems with your adrenal glands?

The adrenals are small glands that sit atop each kidney. As discussed in chapter 1, there are several conditions of the adrenals that can raise blood pressure.

Primary aldosteronism. An overactive adrenal gland can produce an excess of the hormone aldosterone, which raises blood pressure. Low potassium in the blood is a clue to this condition because aldosterone controls the amount of potassium in the body.

Adrenal hyperactivity (Cushing's Syndrome). If the adrenal glands produce too much of the hormone cortisone, the blood pressure will be raised. The clue to this disease is unusual weight gain on the upper back and abdomen. Distinctive violet-colored stretch marks may develop on the abdomen. Blood or urine testing will reveal excess cortisone.

Pheochromocytoma. The cause of high blood pressure here is a tumor of the central part of the adrenal gland, the adrenal medulla. Persons with this problem complain of attacks of headache, sweating, tremor and heart palpitations all at the same time. If you report these symptoms, the doctor may ask you to collect your urine for 24 hours. This is then analyzed for chemicals secreted by the tumor. If this test is positive, then special X-rays are done to locate the tumor, which can often be removed by surgery.

HAS HIGH BLOOD PRESSURE AFFECTED YOUR BODY?

As discussed more fully in chapter 1, if your blood pressure is very high or high for a long time, it can affect the organs of your body. If the doctor finds that your body is showing the effects of high blood pressure, this is important knowledge when deciding about treatment.

The first area to be affected is the heart. Because the heart must work against higher pressure in hypertension, it will eventually become larger. This is detected by an *echocardiogram* (a picture formed by bouncing sound waves off the heart) early on or, when more advanced, by an *electrocardiogram* (a measurement of the changes in the electrical activity of the heart muscle). A chest X-ray can also measure the heart size. If the heart muscle is overworked for a very long time, fluid may back up into the lungs. This is called *congestive heart failure*. The fluid is easily heard when listening over the lungs with a stethoscope, and can be seen on the chest X-ray.

The second area of the body to be affected is the kidneys. Prolonged high blood pressure can wear out the kidneys. This can be detected by a simple blood test, and 24-hour urine collection is often added for more information.

High blood pressure can also affect the blood vessels in the eyes. By looking into the eye with an ophthalmoscope, the doctor can see what is happening to the blood vessels in the body. With severe hypertension, the blood vessels become narrowed and twisted. The vessels can also leak fluid or blood that can be seen as white or red patches on the back of the eye. The doctor will also examine the large blood vessels of the body for narrowing or enlargement due to high blood pressure.

OTHER CONTRIBUTING FACTORS

Hypertension is treated primarily to lower your chance of having a stroke or heart trouble, so your doctor must know about anything else that could increase your chance of having either of these problems. Tell your doctor if members of your close family have had strokes or heart trouble, if you smoke, or if you have diabetes or high blood cholesterol levels. Your doctor may also run tests for diabetes or cholesterol.

QUESTIONS AND ANSWERS

People with high blood pressure usually have many questions about their condition. Here are answers to some of the more common questions that arise.

Why is my blood pressure sometimes higher when I feel fine and I've been taking all my medicines as prescribed?

Blood pressure is constantly going up and down as we go about our activities. As mentioned earlier, it's quite usual for the diastolic pressure to vary by as much as 10 – 20 mmHg, even within a few minutes. Being rushed or anxious can make it even higher for a short time. Sometimes taking a cold or cough remedy may cause the pressure to rise. The pressure can vary from visit to visit because a different arm is used; it's not uncommon to have 5 – 10 mmHg difference between the two arms, so the custom is to use the arm with the higher blood pressure for all visits. Talking while your blood pressure is being taken can also elevate it. Smoking may briefly raise blood pressure. Your blood pressure will seem to be elevated if it's taken when your arm is not comfortably supported. Finally, your blood pressure may increase over time even though you're taking your medication, so the dosage of the medication must be adjusted.

When the doctor is trying to find out whether the high blood pressure has affected my body, why doesn't he ask about headaches?

Unless it's very high, elevated blood pressure has *no* symptoms. People with mild-to-moderate hypertension have the same number and types of headaches as people with normal blood pressure.

Is there a difference between blood pressure measured with a mercury column machine, a machine with a round dial (aneroid), or an electric machine?

Mercury column instruments provide the most accurate and dependable measurement of blood pressure. Little can go wrong with such machines. The dial and electric machines need to be checked regularly for accuracy. As long as the dial machine has been checked, then the blood pressure recorded will be the same as one taken with a mercury machine. Chapter 15 has more information about blood pressure machines.

Do I have high blood pressure if only my diastolic pressure is high?

If your diastolic pressure stays above 90 mmHg on three different occasions over six months, then you have high blood pressure or hypertension. Most often, but not always, your systolic blood pressure will also be high (that is, over 140 mmHg).

We must note here, however, that there is not full agreement among doctors on the need to treat mild hypertension. If the diastolic blood pressure is 90–100 mmHg and there's no evidence of damage to the heart, brain, kidney or major arteries, then other factors will be taken into account in reaching a decision. These factors include other risks such as smoking, gender, diabetes, cholesterol and family history.

The following tables summarize the doctor's examination for high blood pressure. Not all parts are needed for all patients, however.

Table 1
The Doctor's Interview Regarding High Blood Pressure

Question	Looking for	Why?
Are you taking any medications?	Birth control pill, estrogens, cold remedies, diet pills	Easily removed cause
Do you eat licorice daily?	Large amount of licorice	Easily removed cause
How much alcohol do you drink per day?	Average of more than two drinks	Can cause high blood pressure
Do you restrict salt intake?	Salt intake	Reduction may lower blood pressure
Have you been under recent stress?	Recent stress may raise blood pressure	May need to measure blood pressure at less stressful time
Have you recently gained or lost weight?	Recent weight change	Overweight causes high blood pressure; weight loss may suggest thyroid or adrenal medulla hyperactivity

Question	Looking for	Why?
Have you ever had any kidney problems?	Kidney infection, stones, bleeding, trauma	Kidney diseases are the most common causes of hypertension
Have you ever had a heart problem or stroke?	History of heart attack or stroke	Effect of increased blood pressure on body
Have you ever had any temporary loss of vision, numbness or paralysis?	Warning of stroke	Effect of increased blood pressure on brain
Do you have leg pains when walking?	Pain that stops with rest	Arteries of legs affected
Has anyone in your close family had a heart attack or stroke?	Family history	Increased risk of heart attack or stroke
Do you smoke?	Regular smoking	Increased chance of heart and artery trouble and stroke
Do you exercise?	Healthy habits	Reduce overall risk
Do you know your blood cholesterol levels?	Elevation	Additional risk
Do you restrict your intake of fat?	Good diet	Lower heart disease risk

Table 2
The Doctor's Physical Examination

Examination	Looking for	As evidence of
Measure height, weight.	Overweight	Excess weight as possible cause; increased risk
Look into eyes.	Twisted blood vessels, red and white patches	Blood vessels affected by blood pressure
Listen to abdomen, neck, groin.	High-pitched sound	Narrowing of artery to kidney, brain or leg
Look at skin.	Violet stretch marks on abdomen	Adrenal hyperactivity
Measure blood pressure in both arms.	Difference	Coarctation; important for future blood pressure measurement
Take pulse at wrist and groin; take blood pressure in leg.	Delay in pulse at groin; lowered pressure in leg	Narrowing of aorta (coarctation)
Listen to heart.	Abnormal heart sounds	Heart enlargement or failure from high blood pressure
Listen to chest.	Fluid in lungs	Heart failure from high blood pressure
Feel neck.	Pulses; thyroid	Narrowed arteries; thyroid gland disease
Feel feet.	Poor circulation, swelling	Narrowed arteries, heart failure

Table 3
Routine Tests for Patients with High Blood Pressure

Test	Looking for	As evidence of
Urine	Protein, cells, glucose (sugar)	Kidney problems, diabetes mellitus
Blood potassium	Low potassium	Overactive adrenal gland
Blood creatinine or urea	Elevation	Kidney problems
Electro-cardiogram (ECG)	Heart enlargement or previous heart damage	Effect of blood pressure on heart
Chest X-ray (optional)	Heart enlargement	Effect of blood pressure on heart

Table 4
Other Tests that may be Done

Test	Looking for	As evidence of
Blood cholesterol	High cholesterol	Increased risk of heart disease
Blood glucose	High glucose	Diabetes mellitus
Echocardiogram	Enlarged heart or abnormality of heart function	Effect of blood pressure on heart
24-hour urine collection	Elevated adrenal hormones; high protein; high sodium	Overactive adrenal gland; kidney problems; excess salt intake
Renal scan (renogram) or intravenous pyelogram (IVP)	Reduced size or functioning of one kidney	Kidney problem as cause of hypertension
Renal vein renin test	High renin level from one kidney	Narrowed artery to one kidney
Renal arteriogram	Narrowing of blood vessel to one kidney	Renal artery narrowing (stenosis)
Home blood pressure measuring	Lower blood pressures at home	Over-reactive blood pressure in doctor's office (White Coat Syndrome)
Ambulatory blood pressure monitoring	Blood pressure changes with time and activity or medication	Accurate measure of average blood pressure
Blood count	Anemia	May increase systolic blood pressure

3

The Benefits of Treatment

David L. Sackett, M.D., M.Sc.

WHY TREAT HIGH BLOOD PRESSURE?

You've learned from the earlier chapters in this book that high blood pressure is bad for you. It shortens your life and increases your chances of having a heart attack, a stroke, permanent damage to your vision, damage to your kidneys, and even a ballooning (aneurysm) of your biggest artery (the aorta). You've also learned that nearly everyone with hypertension has no symptoms until complications have set in.

This chapter will answer the question: why treat high blood pressure? The answer is simple: because treating high blood pressure decreases your chances of suffering one of its complications! However, because this answer means that you'll have to take medicine, follow a fairly strict diet, or change your lifestyle even though you may feel perfectly well, you deserve an explanation; so we give one here.

EFFECTIVE TREATMENT — HOW TO TELL

How can we tell if a treatment should be prescribed by doctors and accepted by patients? How can we know that it does more good than harm? After all, it wasn't all that long ago that doctors prescribed opium for diabetes. In fact, this was recommended by one of the world's most famous doctors several decades ago, William Osler.

The first U.S. president was also a victim of bad medical advice. He had a severe sore throat and was prescribed "blood-letting." This was a common medical practice in his day and consisted of taking a quantity of blood over a few days to "let the bad humors out." The result was fatal. The treatment was far worse than the disease!

In modern times, health scientists have developed powerful methods for proving whether a new treatment does more good than harm. Rather than relying on testimonials or the advice of famous doctors, health scientists insist that new treatments be tested in special experiments called *randomized clinical trials.*

A randomized clinical trial uses a computer process, similar to tossing a coin, to determine who will receive the treatment being tested. Within a group of patients who agree to help test the new treatment, individuals are assigned to receive either the new treatment (if the "coin" lands heads-up) or an apparently identical, but actually inert, treatment called a *placebo* (if the "coin" lands tails-up). A placebo has no effect whatsoever on a person's health.

The enormous advantage of this random allocation is that it produces two identical groups of patients, one of which receives the active drug while the other receives the placebo. We can be sure at the end of the study that any differences between the two groups must be due to the different treatments. If the group that received the active drug does better (has fewer symptoms, feels healthier, lives longer), researchers can be confident that the drug does more good than harm. We can then make the treatment available to similar patients everywhere.

If, on the other hand, both groups look and feel the same at the end of the trial, then we know either that the drug is not effective or that whatever good it may do is balanced by some bad side effects. When this result occurs, we know that we have to keep looking for a better treatment.

Sometimes the group receiving the active drug actually does worse than the group receiving placebos. Other clinicians and patients must then be warned not to use this treatment.

In randomized trials that involve the testing of drugs, the active and placebo pills are made to look, feel, smell and taste the same. Moreover, in most randomized trials, both the patient and the patient's doctor have agreed not to be told whether the patient is receiving the active treatment or the placebo. Thus, their conclusions about the drug's effectiveness won't be influenced (or *biased*) by knowing which treatment was being received. When both the patient and the doctor are "blind" as to which is being used — active treatment or placebo — the study is called a *double-blind* trial.

WHAT WE HAVE LEARNED FROM RANDOMIZED TRIALS

Randomized clinical trials have proven that several treatments really do more good than harm. Examples of such treatments are the polio vaccine, the coronary bypass operation, and good old ASA for "little strokes" (the transient ischemic attacks mentioned in chapter 1). The results are impressive. Poliomyelitis is now a very rare disease. Thousands of people who would once have been crippled by heart disease are now leading normal lives. Men with little strokes who take ASA are now only half as likely to suffer or die from big strokes.

Randomized clinical trials have also proven that other treatments are worthless or even harmful. One example is the "gastric freeze" for peptic ulcer, a treatment in which super-cooled fluid was circulated through the stomach in an effort to stop the production of stomach acid. Another example is big doses of vitamin C for cancer. A third is the carotid bypass operation to prevent strokes, in which an artery from the scalp is attached to an artery supplying the brain. The result of these important studies is that patients are no longer subjected to these useless treatments. The money, time and effort previously wasted on them can now be put to better use.

RANDOMIZED TRIALS IN HYPERTENSION

Some of the very first randomized clinical trials ever conducted were carried out in the sixties to test whether the treatment of high blood pressure did more good than harm. They involved patients with very severe hypertension. One hundred forty-three men with diastolic blood pressures (diastolic being the lower of the two blood pressure readings, representing the pressure in the large arteries between heartbeats) of between 115 and 129 millimetres of mercury agreed to join this first trial. Seventy were randomly assigned to receive inert pills (placebos). The other 73 were randomly assigned to receive active pills containing drugs that would lower their blood pressure.

During the months that followed, 27 of the 70 men taking the placebos (that is, 39 percent of them) suffered complications of their hypertension such as strokes, severe damage to their eyes, hearts or kidneys, or even death. Over this same time, however, the 73 men taking the active drugs fared much better. Only two of these 73 men (or three percent of them) suffered complications of their hypertension.

As soon as it was clear that this dramatic difference could not be due to chance, the trial was stopped and the men who had been taking the placebos were started on active medicine. We had proof, for the first time, that treating high blood pressure did more good than harm.

But that was only the beginning of the story. We now had proof that the treatment of the most severe form of hypertension was effective. But what about less severe elevations in blood pressure?

RECENT TRIALS IN HYPERTENSION

More randomized clinical trials followed. In each of them, patients with successively smaller elevations in blood pressure agreed to be treated randomly with placebos or active drugs. Every time, the answer was the same: treating high blood pressure does more good than harm.

However, as patients with less and less severe hypertension joined these studies, two additional answers emerged. First, as suggested from earlier community studies (such as the famous Framingham Heart Epidemiology Study), it became clear that the smaller the elevation in blood pressure, the smaller the risk of complications. Second, it became clear that the benefits of treatment were much smaller for people with mild hypertension.

For example, the earliest trials among the most severely hypertensive patients showed us that, without treatment, two out of every three would have a disabling stroke or die within five years. With treatment, we could prevent half of these serious complications, so that only one out of the three would die or have a disabling stroke within five years.

With mild hypertension, the risk of such serious complications is much less. Without treatment, only four of every 200 mild hypertensives suffer a disabling stroke or die within five years. With treatment, we could prevent a quarter of these serious complications, so that only three out of 200 would die or have a disabling stroke within five years. In other words, large numbers of mildly hypertensive patients had to be treated before we found anyone who benefited significantly from treatment.

Unfortunately, we can't tell beforehand which four of these 200 people are the ones destined for stroke or death. We also don't know ahead of time which of these four will be the person who benefits from treatment. Therefore, we must ask all 200 of them to take the treatment. Of course, this also means they must spend the money for the medicine and run the risks, though small, of side effects from the antihypertensive drugs.

It's not surprising, then, that there is vigorous debate among the experts about whether these mildest hypertensive patients should be treated at all, and especially with drugs.

There is agreement, however, about the more severe forms of hypertension. We all agree that anyone with a diastolic blood pressure of 100 mmHg or greater will benefit from treatment, regardless of age. In addition, individuals with smaller elevations (90 - 100 mmHg diastolic) who also show some evidence that the high blood pressure has affected their hearts, brains, eyes or kidneys have been proven to benefit from treatment.

RESEARCH CONTINUES

The search goes on. There are other types of high blood pressure (for example, the form in which only the systolic, but not the diastolic, reading is high) about which we're still ignorant. Whether these other types of high blood pressure should be treated is currently being studied in randomized trials.

We also don't know very much yet about which blood pressure lowering drugs are preferred by patients. Research on this important topic is intense at present. Unfortunately, it's hampered by difficulties in measuring the quality of life of patients. We should know much more in the next few years.

Many patients with high blood pressure, and many of us who treat them, would prefer to use low-salt diets, weight-reduction, special methods of relaxation, or exercise, if these alternatives to drugs could effectively lower blood pressure and prevent the complications of hypertension. Accordingly, recent randomized trials have considered several of these non-drug treatments of hypertension which you can read about in the next two chapters in this book.

CONCLUSION

So, let's end where we began: why treat high blood pressure? — because treating high blood pressure can prevent or reverse most complications of hypertension. We have learned that treating high blood pressure does more good than harm by applying rigorous scientific methods, most notably the randomized clinical trial, to the study of these treatments. Time and time again, randomized trials have proven that people with high blood pressure live longer and healthier lives when their hypertension is detected and treated, and these studies are continuing to provide important answers that will help us improve the treatment of high blood pressure.

4

Diet and High Blood Pressure

Darlene Abbott, R.N., M.Sc., Beverley Whitmore, R.D., and
Arun Chockalingam, Ph.D.

We know that blood pressure is affected by the kinds of food
we eat, although the exact relationship between diet and high
blood pressure remains somewhat controversial. A Canadian
Consensus Conference was held in 1989 to consider the
evidence for and against non-drug approaches in the prevention and treatment of hypertension. A panel of experts re-
viewed the most recent scientific information and then made
recommendations for the public and for those being treated
for high blood pressure. The main focus of this chapter is the
guidelines for people with high blood pressure.

Seven of the most common factors thought to influence
blood pressure are obesity (overweight), sodium (salt), potassium, calcium, alcohol, relaxation/stress management, and
physical exercise. In this chapter, we'll outline the recommendations on dietary factors and describe the role that diet plays
in prevention and control of high blood pressure. We'll also
provide some practical advice on how to select a healthy diet
and adopt a healthy lifestyle.

All of the information in this chapter must be considered in the broader sense of preventing heart disease. This means that stopping smoking and reducing your blood cholesterol are encouraged, although we won't discuss these factors in detail because they don't affect blood pressure. Other aspects of lifestyle also affect blood pressure, including alcohol, exercise and relaxation. You'll find more information on these in chapter 5.

CANADA'S FOOD GUIDE

Before discussing diet changes that can lower blood pressure, we must start with some basic concepts about food. Canada's Food Guide is considered the best reference on which to pattern your eating habits. This guide, designed by Health and Welfare Canada for Canadians over two years of age, helps you to make sensible and healthy food choices for your body's needs. The guide uses three principles in establishing healthy eating habits: variety (in food choices and eating patterns); a balance between energy intake and energy output; and moderation (in the use of fat, sugar, salt and alcohol).

The guide outlines the four classes of foods and the minimum amount required for a healthy diet. Look at the guide when reviewing your present intake and when considering the recommendations we'll describe concerning high blood pressure. In this way, you can adapt Canada's Food Guide to meet your own needs.

Canada's Food Guide provides 4000 - 6000 kilojoules per day (1000 - 1400 calories) as a basic diet. Most Canadians require more energy than this, and can increase the number or size of servings from the various food groups or add other foods not mentioned in the guide.

Following Canada's Food Guide leads to sensible eating and promotes good health. Good eating habits also help your blood pressure, as we'll explain in this chapter.

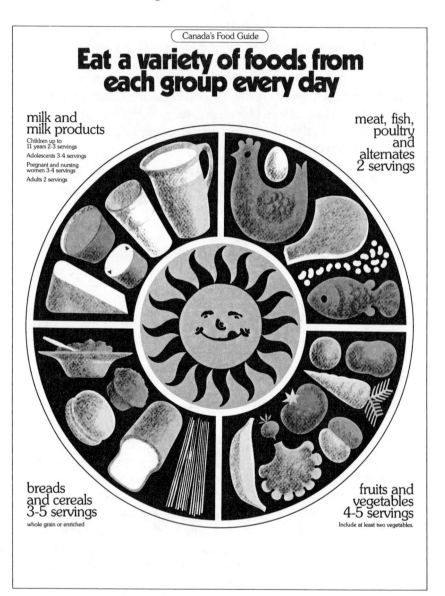

**Figure 1: Canada's Food Guide. (Reproduced with permission of
the Minister of Supply and Services Canada.)**

(Canada's Food Guide)

Variety

Choose different kinds of foods from within each group in appropriate numbers of servings and portion sizes.

Energy Balance

Needs vary with age, sex and activity. Balance energy intake from foods with energy output from physical activity to control weight. Foods selected according to the Guide can supply 4000 – 6000 kJ (kilojoules) (1000 – 1400 kilocalories). For additional energy, increase the number and size of servings from the various food groups and/or add other foods.

Moderation

Select and prepare foods with limited amounts of fat, sugar and salt. If alcohol is consumed, use limited amounts.

milk and milk products

Children up to 11 years	**2-3 servings**
Adolescents	**3-4 servings**
Pregnant and nursing women	**3-4 servings**
Adults	**2 servings**

Skim, 2%, whole, buttermilk, reconstituted dry or evaporated milk may be used as a beverage or as the main ingredient in other foods. Cheese may also be chosen.

Some examples of one serving
250 mL (1 cup) milk
175 mL (¾ cup) yoghurt
45 g (1½ ounces) cheddar or process cheese

In addition, a supplement of vitamin D is recommended when milk is consumed which does not contain added vitamin D.

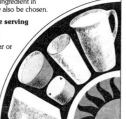

meat, fish, poultry and alternates
2 servings

Some examples of one serving
60 to 90 g (2–3 ounces) cooked lean meat, fish, poultry or liver
60 mL (4 tablespoons) peanut butter
250 mL (1 cup) cooked dried peas, beans or lentils
125 mL (½ cup) nuts or seeds
60 g (2 ounces) cheddar cheese
125 mL (½ cup) cottage cheese
2 eggs

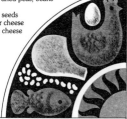

breads and cereals
3-5 servings

whole grain or enriched. Whole grain products are recommended.

Some examples of one serving
1 slice bread
125 mL (½ cup) cooked cereal
175 mL (¾ cup) ready-to-eat cereal
1 roll or muffin
125 to 175 mL (½ – ¾ cup) cooked rice, macaroni, spaghetti or noodles
½ hamburger or wiener bun

fruits and vegetables
4-5 servings

Include at least two vegetables.

Choose a variety of both vegetables and fruits — cooked, raw or their juices. Include yellow, green or green leafy vegetables.

Some examples of one serving
125 mL (½ cup) vegetables or fruits – fresh, frozen or canned
125 mL (½ cup) juice – fresh, frozen or canned
1 medium-sized potato, carrot, tomato, peach, apple, orange or banana

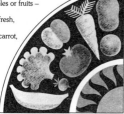

OBESITY

When people gain weight, their blood pressure often rises. High blood pressure occurs about twice as often in persons who are overweight as in those who are not. Weight gain that occurs during early adult life appears to increase the chances of developing hypertension in later years. In fact, young adults who are overweight are five times more likely to develop high blood pressure than those who have a healthy body weight. Family history also plays a role. Studies show that young people who are overweight and have at least one parent with high blood pressure are at even greater risk of becoming hypertensive.

There's also some evidence that certain overweight people are at greater risk than others. For example, recent research has shown that people who have their fat concentrated in the upper part of the body (that is, waist and abdomen) are more prone to high blood pressure than if the excess fat is located on the thighs or buttocks.

Most important, when people lose weight their blood pressure may fall. Weight loss has also been found to lower blood pressure effectively in patients being treated for hypertension. This effect is more dramatic in the obese, but reductions in blood pressure have been noted even in those people not considered to be overweight.

How much weight must you lose to reduce your blood pressure? — this will vary with the individual. While it makes good sense to aim for a healthy body weight, you may not have to achieve this goal to lower your blood pressure. Blood pressures may fall as long as there is a sustained weight loss. For example, losing five kilograms may lower your blood pressure by six to ten millimetres of mercury, even though you may still be considered overweight. This is an important point to remember if your doctor has prescribed weight loss as a way of controlling your blood pressure. You and your doctor will have to watch the changes in your blood pressure as you lose weight.

We must note here that weight loss does not always result in lower blood pressure, just as being overweight does not always mean that your blood pressure will be elevated. However, losing excess weight has other benefits even if your blood pressure is not reduced.

Before we tell you how to lose weight sensibly, it might be helpful to know whether or not you need to lose weight. You can do this by determining your body mass index (BMI), using the chart on page 62. Note that the BMI includes weight from all body sources, including fat. This index applies only to adults 20 – 65 years of age, and doesn't make allowances for increased muscle mass (for example, in athletes) or distribution of body fat. Thus, it's only a guideline. You and your doctor should discuss what weight is healthiest for you.

Based on the evidence, the Canadian Consensus Conference recommended that all adult Canadians aim for a BMI of 20 to 27, and that all overweight persons being treated for hypertension reduce their weight. Sensible weight loss and, more important, maintaining a healthy body weight are achieved by restricting calories in combination with regular exercise.

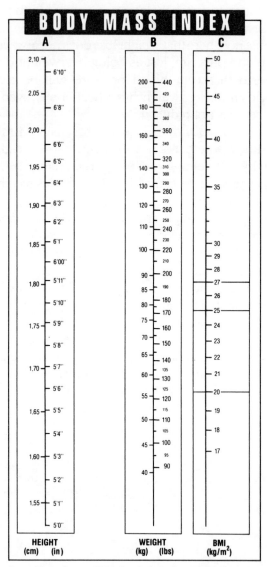

Source: Expert Group on Weight Standards, Health and Welfare Canada

**Figure 2: Calculating your BMI. (Reprinted with permission
from the Canadian Dietetic Association.)**

Sensible weight control

Anyone who has tried to lose weight knows that it can be both difficult and frustrating. Many people resort to fad diets that promise quick, easy weight loss. While these diets may result in some weight loss, it seldom lasts. Nor does this approach provide adequate nutrition for good health. Making healthier food choices and exercising more often are the best ways to lose weight and keep it off.

When the amount of energy you put out is greater than the amount of calories you take in, you create a negative balance and lose weight. One way to learn about this balance is to record *everything* you eat and drink for a minimum of four days. At the same time, record all activities you engage in (for example, sitting at your desk, driving, gardening, doing housework, and so on). Be honest with yourself. This is a good way to learn more about your present lifestyle and your eating habits.

When you have completed your record, use the following steps to find out if you are eating sensibly:

1. Look at the basic foods from each food group in the amounts recommended in Canada's Food Guide. Compare this to the amount of food you have recorded. For example (recorded intake of breakfast):

125 mL (1/2 cup) orange juice	= 1 fruit serving
1 slice brown toast	= 1 bread or cereal serving
5 mL (1 tsp) butter	= no food group
5 mL (1 tsp) jam	= no food group
250 mL (1 cup) milk	= 1 milk serving

2. Do you have all the recommended servings from Canada's Food Guide? Is there any group in which you are consis-

tently short? If so, how can you increase your intake? Do you usually eat more from one food group than is required? How can you reduce the intake of this food group in your daily eating habits?

3. Look at the foods you ate that don't fit into any of the four food groups. These foods are often high in calories and have little food value. Could you decrease or omit them from your diet?

4. How often are you eating apart from regular meals? Do you try to have three regular meals per day or do you snack throughout the day? Snacking can be a habit or a way of coping with stress. If your snacks are good food choices and don't affect your weight, it may not be necessary to stop them.

5. Are you able to do some form of regular exercise during the week, such as walking? How often are you able to do this?

The key to losing weight and keeping it off is a consistently healthy diet. Chronic dieting, and fluctuations between weight loss and weight gain, can have serious effects on your health and make it harder for you to lose weight. Diet sensibly. Plan your meals around Canada's Food Guide, eat regular meals, and gradually increase your exercise. (It's a good idea to check with your doctor before you start exercising.) Take your time and make realistic changes in your eating habits. Ask your family to help you make these changes.

A safe weight loss is considered to be in the range of one-half to one kilogram (one to two pounds) a week. If you can't achieve this using the above guidelines, ask your doctor to refer you to a dietitian. You may also need some professional advice on an exercise program.

SALT

Salt and *sodium* are used interchangeably throughout this chapter.

For some time now, it has been thought that salt plays an important role in the development of high blood pressure. Evidence to support this theory comes mostly from studying different populations. The results have shown that undeveloped societies have a low sodium intake and a low incidence of high blood pressure. Industrialized societies, however, have a high intake of sodium and have higher rates of hypertension.

Both hypertension and salt intake increase as a society modernizes. What is not so clear, however, is whether high salt intake causes hypertension. For example, the tribal Indians in Brazil eat very little salt and have little or no incidence of high blood pressure. But these people are usually thin, physically active, drink no alcohol, and live in a relatively stress-free environment. Their lifestyle is not exactly comparable to that of most North Americans!

A wide-ranging study known as INTERSALT was undertaken to settle, once and for all, whether salt is related to blood pressure. INTERSALT involved 32 countries from Argentina to Iceland, from Mexico to Zimbabwe, and included ten thousand people. The INTERSALT results did show that blood pressure tends to be higher among people who consume more salt. However, the overall effect was quite small, particularly on the diastolic pressure. What seemed to be more closely related to lower blood pressure was the dietary combination of a lower salt intake and a higher potassium intake. Such diets also tended to be lower in calories, so perhaps lower weight also contributes to the positive effect.

The researchers concluded that the dietary changes normally found in a low-salt diet (that is, low calories and high potassium) could potentially result in a drop of blood pressure averaging two to three millimetres of mercury. Even this small drop in blood pressure would have a positive effect on the general population and would reduce the overall incidence of hypertension.

The best way to test the effect of lower salt is to do a randomized trial (as described in chapter 3). In such a trial, people with untreated high blood pressure would be given either a low-salt diet or a normal-salt diet, and then the blood pressures of the two groups would be followed. There have been several trials like this. One review of these studies found that some trials showed a significant effect from the low-salt diet, but even more showed no benefit. In view of this situation, it's difficult to make a firm recommendation.

The studies just mentioned were among people not taking medication for their high blood pressure. Among people on medication, sodium restriction has been found to enhance the effects of most drugs; one exception is that salt restriction does not seem to increase the effect of calcium antagonists (these antihypertensive drugs are described in chapter 10).

We've seen that studies of salt restriction among people on no medication give conflicting results. One explanation is that some people may be salt sensitive. At present, there's no practical way of knowing who responds to salt and who doesn't. However, if you're on medication, salt restriction may reduce the amount of medication required to keep your blood pressure under control. In addition, it makes good health sense to decrease the amount of salt you consume. Sodium intake of Canadians far exceeds the amount required for their daily needs. Recent studies have found that 15 percent of our daily sodium intake comes from cooking and adding salt at the table. The rest comes primarily from processed and "fast" foods, with about 10 percent being naturally present in food. Thus, you must pay attention to the amount of salt that's already in the food you buy.

How to reduce the salt in your diet

The taste preference for salt is an acquired habit and will go away after a few months of restricting intake. Set aside three to six months and slowly decrease your salt intake. This should be a more tolerable way for you to make long-lasting changes in your diet.

The first step is to avoid adding salt to food served at the table. Once the food without added salt tastes acceptable to you, begin to analyze your food purchasing patterns. This means that you should choose fresh or frozen foods rather than canned or packaged items. Make a practice of reading food labels. Ingredients are listed in order of the amount found in the product. For example, this passage is taken from a package label: "Frozen Chicken Nuggets — this product contains chicken, *salt,* lemon juice, spices. Bread crumb coating contains modified starch, wheat flour, corn flour, *salt,* hydrogenated vegetable oil, *baking powder,* soy flour, milk solids, dried egg white, spices, guar gum, and *monosodium glutamate.*"

The point in reading labels is to avoid salt or sodium compounds found in food products (in this example they've been italized). If any of these are listed near the beginning, or if there are three or more sodium sources listed in the product, then you should avoid buying it. Judging from the example, frozen chicken nuggets would not be a good product to buy.

Items for you to avoid when shopping for groceries include: processed meats such as bologna, sausages, hot dogs; smoked meats such as corned beef; processed cheeses, pickles, canned or dried soup mixes; regular canned vegetables or vegetable juice; salted nuts, seasoning salts, and most prepared sauces or dressings.

Foods that you should buy include: fresh or frozen vegetables, milk and milk products, lean meats, whole-grain enriched breads, and cereal products.

Decreasing your salt intake slowly will allow you to get used to the taste of natural foods. You may be surprised by how good a fresh tomato tastes without salt! If you want to add flavor to your foods, use herbs and spices. A low-salt cookbook will provide you with many ideas, but here are a few suggestions:

- Ground beef: chili powder, oregano, allspice, basil, savory, rosemary.

- Roast chicken: rub well inside and out with a mixture of salad oil and ginger before roasting.

- Potatoes: parsley, mace, chopped green pepper, onion, rosemary (added to water during cooking).

For more suggestions on how to use flavorings, contact your local dietitian or the Heart and Stroke Foundation.

POTASSIUM

There's some evidence that populations consuming foods high in potassium have lower blood pressures. But a diet rich in potassium is, by its very nature, also low in sodium. It's probably the combination of a low-sodium and a high-potassium diet that's most important in preventing the development of hypertension.

High-potassium diets have been found to lower blood pressures in some individuals being treated for hypertension. Some studies have used potassium pills as a way of increasing potassium in the body. These have also been found to reduce blood pressure, although the studies have followed patients for only a short time. A potassium-rich diet is especially important for people who are taking certain diuretics (water pills) for their high blood pressure, because these pills deplete the body of potassium.

The typical North American diet contains only one-quarter as much potassium as people have eaten throughout history. Increasing the amount of potassium we now eat will certainly not harm us. (NOTE: People with kidney disease should not alter their potassium intake before discussing this with their doctors.) A potassium-rich diet, in combination with a low-salt diet, is especially recommended for those individuals being treated with thiazide diuretics (discussed in chapter 7).

How to get enough potassium into your daily diet

Contrary to what you may have heard, you don't have to eat a bunch of bananas a day or drink litres of orange juice to get enough potassium! If you follow Canada's Food Guide, you'll get the amount required for good health. If, for some reason, your body can't maintain an adequate level of potassium (for example, certain diseases and some medications can cause you to lose potassium), you may have to increase the amount of potassium-rich foods you eat. Check with your doctor to find out what's best for you.

As well as eating foods from all four food groups, you can increase your potassium intake by preparing foods in certain ways. Cooking food in a lot of water removes potassium. This can be prevented by leaving the skins on vegetables, cutting food into large pieces when boiling, and cooking until just tender in a small amount of water. Try steaming or baking your vegetables, or use a microwave oven. A baked potato is high in potassium.

The following table provides some examples of excellent sources of potassium.

Table 1: Foods high in potassium.

EXCELLENT SOURCES
(at least 500 mg per serving)

Meat and alternates

Peas and beans
250 ml (1 cup)
Chick peas, split peas, common white beans, lima beans, red kidney beans, soy beans

Nuts and seeds
125 ml (1/2 cup)
Almonds and peanuts (shelled), sunflower seeds

Fruits and vegetables

Vegetables
250 ml (1 cup)
Beet greens, parsnips, pumpkin, spinach, winter squash, tomato or vegetable juice

1 medium (100 g)
Potato baked in skin

Fruits

125 ml (1/2 cup)	Seedless raisins
250 ml (1 cup)	Orange or prune juice, rhubarb
1/2 medium (142 g)	Avocado
1/2 medium (385 g)	Cantaloup or honeydew melon
1 medium (175 g)	Banana
1 medium (304 g)	Papaya
1 slice (925 g)	Watermelon
5 halves (72 g)	Dried peaches
10 halves (79 g)	Dried apricots
10 medium (100 g)	Pitted dates

Milk

250 ml (1 cup)
Whole, two percent, skim, reconstituted skim (25 g powder = 250 ml), goat milk, buttermilk

(Adapted from *Foods High in Potassium* with permission from Calgary

---

GOOD SOURCES
(300–500 mg per serving)

Meat and alternates

Meat, liver, fish
90 g (3 oz)

Any cut of lean beef or pork, cod, halibut, salmon, scallops, sardines

Lentils and nuts
250 ml (1 cup)   Lentils
125 ml (1/2 cup)   Brazil nuts, cashews, pecans
15 ml (1 tbsp)   Peanut butter

Fruits and vegetables

Vegetables
250 ml (1 cup)

Beets, broccoli, brussels sprouts, carrots, cauliflower, celery, eggplant, mushrooms, summer squash, turnips, tomatoes, zucchini

100 g (1 medium)   Sweet potato, peeled and boiled potato

Fruits
250 ml (1 cup)   Apricot nectar, grapefruit or pineapple
                        or tangerine juice
241 g (1/2 medium)   Grapefruit
150 g (1 medium)   Orange

Health Services.)

CALCIUM

Although there has been some evidence to suggest that dietary calcium can affect blood pressure, we can't say for sure that increased calcium intake will prevent high blood pressure. Nor does calcium supplementation (food or pills) lower blood pressure in people being treated for hypertension. As the association between calcium and high blood pressure is inconclusive, no specific recommendations were made by the panel at the Consensus Conference.

The calcium/high blood pressure theory does have potential, though, and studies are under way in Canada to explore the connection. For now, the best advice is to follow Canada's Food Guide to be sure you get an adequate amount of calcium in your diet. Because many people don't eat enough calcium-rich foods, some calcium supplementation may be helpful in preventing other conditions, such as osteoporosis. (Osteoporosis is a weakening and brittleness of the bones, found in some post-menopausal women.)

CHOLESTEROL

Do you know your cholesterol level? The level of cholesterol in your blood doesn't affect your blood pressure. However, high blood cholesterol increases the chances of developing heart disease, so it's important to control your cholesterol level as well as your high blood pressure. More details on a low-cholesterol diet can be obtained from your doctor, through referral to a dietitian, or from the Heart and Stroke Foundation.

MENU PLANNING AND RESTAURANT MEALS

Time is a precious commodity today, which adds to the challenge of meal preparation. The result is an increasing consumption of "convenience" foods from both the grocery store and from fast-food restaurants. These meals tend to be high in salt, fat and calories, and may not be suitable for someone who has high blood pressure.

If you find that you're eating convenience foods often, ask yourself some questions: Do you enjoy these meals? Are they really saving you time? Have you ever stopped to calculate the cost of these convenience meals? Is this a healthy diet? If you answered no to any of these questions, you probably need to make some changes in your food purchases.

First, do some menu planning (for a week at a time). This may take only 15 minutes. It doesn't have to be detailed. Plan meals that are simple and quick to prepare. Then, make a grocery list from your menu so you can have all the ingredients on hand. Finally, involve all members of the family in meal preparation. Children will often eat better when they have helped prepare a meal. Here are a few fast dinner ideas:

- Tip: Roast beef, chicken or turkey on Sunday; have cold sliced meat for Monday.

  Menu: Cold roast beef/baked potato/raw vegetables/ fresh fruit/milk

- Tip: Homemade spaghetti sauce can be made in bulk and frozen in meal-sized containers.

  Menu: Spaghetti/sauce/salad/fresh bread/fruit/milk

- Tip: Put stew meat and vegetables in crock pot in the morning.

  Menu: Stew/fresh buns/fruit/milk

- Tip: Use slices of chicken, beef or pork in preparation of stir fries.

  Menu: Stir-fried meats and vegetables/rice or noodles/fresh fruit/milk

- Tip: Use your microwave.

  Menu: Fish/baked potato/frozen vegetables/low-fat frozen yogurt/milk

If you're eating out, here are some tips for enjoying a healthy restaurant meal:

- Anticipate what the menu will be when choosing a restaurant; for example, a fish 'n' chips restaurant will offer few options.

- Avoid buffets, which encourage overeating.

- Eat slowly until you're comfortably full; you don't have to eat everything on your plate.

- Select foods without cream sauces, gravies, etc.; a broiled steak or baked fish with a lemon wedge would be a good choice.

- Choose food that has been prepared by broiling, steaming, or poaching.

• Enjoy other aspects of the meal besides food, including the atmosphere, the company and the relaxation associated with eating out.

ALCOHOL

Alcohol and high blood pressure are discussed in chapter 5, but we'll briefly review them here. There's convincing evidence that drinking alcohol increases blood pressure. This can lead to the development of high blood pressure in some individuals and may worsen the blood pressure in those who already have hypertension. This is true for both men and women.

You should limit your daily drinking to no more than two *standard drinks*. A standard drink is 120 ml (4 oz) of wine, or 30 ml (1oz) of liquor, or 360 ml (12 oz) of beer. If you have hypertension that is not controlled, the Canadian Consensus Conference recommended that you may need to cut out drinking alcoholic beverages altogether.

One more word of advice: avoid binge drinking, as this has been found to increase the incidence of stroke. This is one risk you want to avoid, even if you have normal blood pressure.

CONCLUSIONS

Diet and lifestyle factors play an important part in the prevention and control of hypertension. Reduction of alcohol intake and weight loss (in combination with increased physical activity) are considered to be effective ways of lowering blood pressure. Although the effect of salt restriction and increased potassium on blood pressure may be small, reducing salt intake also enhances the effect of most drugs used in the treatment of high blood pressure.

Eating the right kinds of foods isn't difficult. Many of the dietary factors discussed tend to be linked. For example, a high-potassium diet will tend to be low in salt and low in cholesterol. Similarly, a restricted-calorie diet will be lower in salt. These natural combinations make it easier to make healthy food choices.

The value of dietary changes varies from person to person. You and your doctor will need to work together to decide on the best approach for you.

5

Lifestyle and High Blood Pressure

Jane Irvine, D.Phil. and Jean Cleroux, Ph.D.

RISK FACTORS FOR HYPERTENSION

As mentioned earlier, the cause of someone's hypertension can't be determined in about 95 percent of cases. High blood pressure of unknown cause is termed *essential hypertension*. Lifestyle — how we eat, drink, exercise and handle stress — does appear, however, to influence the development of essential hypertension. These influences are called *risk factors* because they appear to be related to developing the disorder and may aggravate hypertension once it sets in. More important, reducing or eliminating some of these lifestyle risk factors may lower blood pressure.

Diet and weight are perhaps the most important influences, and they're discussed in chapter 4. In this chapter, we'll describe the ways that alcohol, stress and exercise are related to blood pressure. We'll then discuss the prospects for lowering your blood pressure by improving these aspects of your lifestyle.

Alcohol

Numerous studies have shown that the more alcohol is consumed, the higher the blood pressure and the more likely the development of hypertension. However, there's some uncertainty about just how alcohol affects blood pressure. One group of reports suggests that the effect of alcohol begins with very small amounts, and that people who don't drink alcohol have the lowest blood pressures. However, a second group of reports shows that one or two alcoholic drinks a day have little effect, but three or more drinks a day is associated with progressively higher blood pressure. Finally, there are a few studies reporting that people who have one or two alcoholic drinks a day have lower blood pressures than either those who abstain or those who have more than three alcoholic drinks a day. In other words, taking three or more drinks per day is certainly harmful, but it's unclear whether consumption below this level affects blood pressure.

It's also interesting that one or two drinks per day raise the amount of "high-density lipoprotein" cholesterol. This is the "good" form of cholesterol that reduces the risk of *coronary heart disease* (damage to the blood vessels that surround and feed the heart muscle). Thus, from the perspective of hypertension and atherosclerosis at least, one to two alcoholic drinks per day may actually be beneficial.

By the way, there's no proof that one *type* of alcoholic beverage is better for your blood pressure than another; what matters is the total *amount* of alcohol consumed. Furthermore, common sense dictates that even the consumption of one or two drinks a day could be dangerous before driving a vehicle, when operating machinery, or in other situations requiring sharp wits and reflexes.

Smoking

Smoking (or chewing) tobacco is not a cause of hypertension. There is, however, a temporary increase in blood pressure (by about 10 mmHg systolic pressure and 8 mmHg diastolic pressure) while smoking and shortly thereafter. Even more important, smoking appears to cancel the beneficial effects of some antihypertensive medications. For example, one large trial found that beta-blockers (a type of medication that lowers blood pressure; see chapter 8) decreased the risk of heart disease and stroke only in those hypertensives who didn't smoke. Furthermore, smoking is one of the most important risk factors for coronary heart disease, stroke and cancer. Risk factors are additive: if you both smoke and have hypertension, you're at even greater risk of heart disease and stroke.

Stress

Does acute stress raise blood pressure? There's a well-known response of the body to acute (short-term) stress termed the *alarm reaction*, the *defence reaction* or the *fight-or-flight response*. This is characterized by an increase in blood pressure, heart rate, respiratory (breathing) rate and muscle tension. There's also an increase in blood flow to the skeletal muscles and a decrease in blood flow to the skin, kidneys and bowels. Hormones such as adrenaline and nor-adrenaline are released into the blood and in turn increase the stimulation to the body.

This reaction is natural and healthy, and it helps the body to respond to danger. The response may be inappropriate, however, if it occurs when no course of action is possible. In other words, if this alarm response is not followed by some action such as fighting or fleeing, then the body is aroused beyond what's required.

The alarm response is usually short-lived, decreasing rapidly when the stress is over. However, it may be harmful in individuals who have either a family history of hypertension or an existing cardiovascular disease. In these individuals, the increase in blood pressure tends to be greater and more prolonged.

Is chronic stress associated with hypertension? In some situations, a chronic (long-term) state of alarm has been associated with high blood pressure. For example, hypertension was found to be more common among people exposed to combat during the Second World War and among men anticipating unemployment, showing that certain stressful conditions can produce a sustained elevation in blood pressure. In these studies, however, blood pressure returned to normal once conditions returned to normal.

If stressful conditions were more prolonged, would the increase in blood pressure become permanent, persisting even when the stress was removed? Researchers have studied people exposed to long-term stressful conditions. These studies have found a higher likelihood of hypertension in certain job conditions. For example, higher blood pressures were found among air traffic controllers and among manual or machine workers who reported that their superiors were generally unsupportive. Working or living in very noisy conditions has been linked with higher rates of hypertension. High blood pressure is also more common in individuals who reside in high-stress neighborhoods where income is low while crime rates, marital breakup rates, the number of residents and resident instability are high.

These studies provide some evidence that chronic stress is related to hypertension, but they don't explain why. Is it explained by the acute stress reaction and its associated increase in adrenaline or noradrenaline? Or do other risk factors, such as high rates of alcohol consumption due to stress, account for the relationship between stress and hypertension? As yet, we don't have answers to these questions.

Just the same, most people exposed to stress don't develop hypertension. This finding has led to the theory that individuals may differ in their sensitivity to the effects of stress.

Individual sensitivity to stress. Both genetic (inherited) and personality factors have been studied to see why only some people develop hypertension when under stress. There's good evidence that a family history of hypertension makes the individual prone to react with exaggerated increases in blood pressure when stressed. However, we don't know yet if this exaggerated reaction leads to a permanent increase in blood pressure.

So far, no link has been established between personality factors, such as anger or anxiety, and development of hypertension. Studies of individuals who aren't aware that they have hypertension have found that these unaware hypertensives are no more anxious or angry than individuals who have normal levels of blood pressure.

Does hypertension cause stress? This is an important question. Many people with high blood pressure who feel that they're under stress may be reacting to the discovery of their hypertension. As mentioned above, recent studies show that hypertensive individuals who were unaware of their hypertension did not score higher on tests of anxiety and anger. Rather, higher anxiety and anger scores were found to occur only in hypertensives who knew about their condition. Therefore, it appears that many hypertensive individuals, upon learning about their hypertension, become anxious and angry.

Learning about one's hypertension has also been associated with other problems, including increased work absenteeism, decreased time spent in social/leisure activities, decreased earnings, increased worry about health and increased physical symptoms such as headaches. Health professionals are becoming more aware of these adverse psychological effects, and are helping patients to understand hypertension better and to worry less.

The best way of reducing the effects of learning about one's hypertension appears to be effective blood pressure treatment. Patients whose blood pressures are well controlled by medication appear to suffer fewer problems. If you recognize some of these problems in yourself, remember that they may be due to your concern about your blood pressure. Overcoming them begins with the recognition that effective treatment eliminates almost all of the health risk due to hypertension. If your blood pressure is well controlled, you can lead a normal life in almost every way. Be sure to raise any concerns you may have with your doctor so he can help you.

Exercise

In the 1930s, it was found that athletes had lower blood pressure than people who didn't exercise regularly. This raised the possibility that exercise might lead to decreased blood pressures in hypertensive patients. The first studies compared the incidence of hypertension in physically active and inactive people. Although many such studies showed that average blood pressure (the blood pressure for the whole group) was lower in active workers than in sedentary (i.e., inactive) workers, the incidence of hypertension was found to be similar in both groups. These results couldn't support the theory that exercise decreases the occurrence of hypertension. However, the interpretation of these findings is complicated. For example, hypertension was found more often in individuals whose work involved greater attention, despite their amount of physical activity.

The first indirect evidence of a relationship between the level of physical activity and the later development of hypertension came in the late 1960s and 1970s. Researchers found that the incidence of hypertension in people who had participated in at least five hours of sports activities per week during their college years was 20 to 40 percent lower than in people who were less active in their younger years. Moreover, those who had slower heart rates when in college (exercise slows the heart rate at rest) were also less likely to have hypertension 20 to 30 years later. This finding, together with the recent report that slowing the heart rate in animals can retard atherosclerosis (clogging of the arteries), suggests that exercise may be beneficial in several ways. This view is supported by the results of a study published in 1986: it showed that active people live longer even when high blood pressure, smoking and obesity are taken into account.

In other studies, the heart function of hypertensive individuals was examined during exercise. These studies showed that abnormalities of the heart occurred less often in physically active people than in sedentary hypertensive people.

These findings are encouraging because they indicate that being physically active may lessen your chance of becoming hypertensive or of having an abnormal reaction during exercise if you're already hypertensive. However, they don't show that becoming more physically active can reverse the changes. To determine if exercise can be of any value in the treatment of hypertension, a given group of previously inactive hypertensive individuals must be submitted to an exercise program and its effects on blood pressure levels examined. We'll briefly summarize the results from such studies later in this chapter. We'll also give practical recommendations about exercise.

MODIFYING YOUR LIFESTYLE

If certain lifestyle factors increase the risk of developing hypertension, then changing these factors may help prevent it, or decrease the blood pressure if it's already elevated. In the following sections, we'll focus on methods to modify alcohol consumption, stress, and physical activity.

Alcohol

Recommendations about alcohol. Based on the evidence relating alcohol consumption to blood pressure, the goal is to drink no more than two standard alcoholic drinks per day. A standard drink is 120 ml (4 oz) of wine, 30 ml (1 oz) of liquor and 360 ml (12 oz) of beer. If your blood pressure is still not controlled, abstinence may be helpful. Also, if you find it difficult to stick to your limit of two standard drinks per day, abstinence may be necessary, at least in the short run, to get you started in changing your drinking patterns.

Alcohol restriction can be tried as a first step in treating mildly elevated blood pressure, that is, a diastolic blood pressure between 90 and 100 mmHg. It's also important to note that other types of antihypertensive treatments are likely to be made less effective if you continue to consume excess alcohol. (For example, stress management has been shown to be less effective in patients who consume alcohol heavily.) The same is likely to apply to antihypertensive medications, diet and exercise.

How to change your drinking patterns and reduce your consumption. To begin changing your drinking pattern, you may find it helpful to keep a record of your drinking behavior, including:

- the number of abstinent days, moderate drinking days (consumed one to four standard drinks, daily), and heavy drinking days (consumed five or more drinks, daily) in a month

- the number of days since your last drink

- the estimated duration of this drinking pattern.

Alcohol consumption usually fits a pattern that serves a function for you. You may drink to reduce feelings of tension or sadness, to have pleasure, to aid some kind of performance (for example, socializing), and to reduce social pressure or be part of the crowd. Sometimes drinking serves no particular purpose; it's just a habit. Alcohol consumption can have one or more functions in the same individual. Understanding the functions alcohol serves for you can help you find alternatives for each function.

Set your own goal. The ultimate goal is to have no more than two standard drinks per day. At first you may want to set a slightly higher goal of, say, three drinks if you are used to drinking quite heavily. However, until you reach no more than two drinks per day, you may not experience much of a blood pressure response. In setting a drinking goal, you should specify your limits:

- your maximum number of drinking days per week

- your maximum number of drinks on drinking days

- when it's all right to drink

- when it's not all right to drink (based on your analysis of your drinking pattern)

- how long you're going to try to change your drinking pattern (i.e., at what point you may want to seek help from an experienced therapist).

You may want to try various strategies to help you reach your goal. One strategy is pacing your drinking, including:

- measuring each drink

- mixing drinks rather than having them straight

- sipping drinks rather than gulping them

- spacing drinks by alternating alcoholic and non-alcoholic drinks or by letting at least one hour pass before taking the next drink

- avoiding drinking on an empty stomach.

Another strategy is self-monitoring of drinking. Self-monitoring includes keeping a record of:

- time of alcohol consumption

- quantity consumed

- reason for drinking

- urges or temptations to drink

- pressures from others to drink.

Self-monitoring will help remind you of your goal, clarify the reasons for your drinking, and identify problem areas.

Decide in advance what you will do when alcohol is freely available (remember the pacing tips) or when pressures from others are likely to occur (e.g., you can remind yourself to say, "Thank you, I'm OK for now"). Set ahead of time the maximum number of drinks you'll consume. Be prepared to counteract your own excuses to go over your goal (e.g., "I'm not working tomorrow", or "I'm not driving tonight").

Take up activities that do not go with heavy drinking. For example, follow an educational or physical fitness program, develop or re-activate a hobby, and change your social network to support your drinking goal.

Problems at home or work may make you feel like drinking. You must set a rule that alcohol should not be used to cope with problems. Find other solutions. You may want to seek help from an experienced therapist for these problems, but often it can help to ask a close friend for advice. If you find that you can't achieve your drinking goal, then you may find it useful to ask your doctor to help plan and supervise the program with you. He can also refer you to an experienced therapist.

Methods for reducing alcohol intake have also been discussed in a self-help pamphlet and manual. If you'd like to have these materials, write to: Dr. Martha Sanchez-Craig, Addiction Research Foundation, 33 Russell Street, Toronto, Ontario M5S 2S1.

Smoking

Recommendations about smoking. It's not easy to quit smoking, but it's particularly important for people with high blood pressure to do so. Many of the tactics discussed for reducing alcohol intake work for cigarette smoking as well. Try them! In addition, there are many helpful aids and programs for quitting. If you find it difficult to stop smoking on your own, your doctor can help you or refer you to special clinics.

Stress

Does relaxation therapy lower blood pressure? When considering the results of relaxation therapy, it's important to recall that blood pressure is extremely variable. We know that blood pressure readings taken in one situation don't always accurately reflect the level of blood pressure in other situations. In fact, numerous studies have found that blood pressures in the doctor's office are not typical of blood pressures at work or home. This difference is important. It means that, although individuals may have learned to relax and lower their blood pressure in the doctor's office, their usual blood pressure may not be lower if they have not learned to relax at work or home.

Even in the clinic, the results of studies of relaxation therapy often disagree. To give you a flavor of the evidence — so you can make your own decision about trying relaxation techniques — we'll review some of the better studies.

Four of seven studies with drug-free hypertensive patients have reported significant decreases in blood pressures that were measured in the clinic. The blood pressure reductions were quite variable. Some patients showed a large fall in blood pressure but others had only small or no change in blood pressure. On average, there was a reduction in systolic pressure of 12 mmHg and diastolic pressure of 10 mmHg.

Nine of 14 studies found relaxation therapy to significantly lower blood pressure among patients who were taking antihypertensive medications but whose blood pressures were still elevated. Another recent study found that many hypertensive patients could reduce the amount of medication taken after relaxation therapy and still maintain good blood pressure control.

It's less certain whether relaxation therapy reduces blood pressure outside the clinic. Two studies have found that blood pressures measured during the work day were lower following relaxation therapy. Another study did not find that blood pressures measured during the work day were lower following relaxation therapy. Therefore, it's still uncertain whether or not relaxation therapy does lower blood pressure over the whole day.

Recommendations regarding relaxation therapy. Relaxation therapy can't be confidently recommended as a treatment for hypertension. First, it's not certain whether relaxation therapy lowers blood pressure over the whole day. Second, there have been no studies to determine if relaxation therapy can prevent hypertensive-related complications such as heart disease and stroke. Thus, the recommendation of a recent Canadian Consensus Conference, co-sponsored by the Canadian Hypertension Society, is that it's premature to recommend the use of relaxation/stress management techniques in the treatment of high blood pressure. Nevertheless, some people may experience a fall in blood pressure. Therefore, we recommend that if you try relaxation therapy you do so with the agreement and supervision of your doctor.

Exercise

Exercise to regulate blood pressure. For this discussion, exercise is defined as the regular practice — three times a week — of dynamic (what we often call *aerobic*) exercises. These include jogging, bicycling, aerobic dancing, swimming, and so on. To have an effect, these must be performed above a minimal intensity for an adequate length of time. Minimal intensity varies from person to person and should be determined by an exercise specialist. A typical exercise session might be 40–60 minutes.

This is in contrast to *isometric* exercises such as those performed on muscle building machines or during weight lifting. Research on the effects of isometric exercise training in hypertension is sparse. During both dynamic and isometric exercise blood pressure normally increases. However, it increases much more during isometric than dynamic exercise. Isometric exercises are thus strongly discouraged unless performed in closely supervised conditions. (It would be wise to avoid pushing your car if it's stuck in the snow!)

Results from experimental studies. The recent Consensus Conference considered the role of exercise in controlling hypertension, and made the following recommendations:

> *Individuals with high blood pressure should consult their doctors prior to undertaking strenuous exercise. Appropriate physical activity is a useful part of weight management in the control of high blood pressure. While there is evidence that regular aerobic activity may result in the lowering of blood pressure in clients with mild hypertension, definitive recommendations must await further research to determine the intensity, frequency and duration of the activity required to lower blood pressure, and to determine how long the benefits can be maintained. Activities such as weight lifting are not recommended for hypertensive patients.*

These recommendations are based on findings from experimental studies that have been performed since the late 1960s to examine the possibility that exercise might reduce resting blood pressure in hypertensive individuals. The following observations stand out from the studies performed on the effects of training with dynamic exercises: in hypertensive individuals with blood pressure levels between 140/90 and 150/100 mmHg, a decrease in resting blood pressure was usually reported after training; in hypertensive individuals with blood pressure levels above 160/100 mmHg, a decrease in resting blood pressure was reported only when the relative intensity of exercise performed was moderate, not when it was higher.

It's beyond the scope of this discussion to define precisely what is meant by "moderate" or "higher" exercise performance. Briefly put, exercise intensity that may be exhausting for one individual could easily be tolerated by another. How to rate the intensity of a particular exercise requires extensive knowledge of physiological processes and should be left to the judgment of exercise specialists.

One important question about exercise is whether the blood pressure lowering effect can be preserved as long as the training regimen is maintained. Little data is available on this point. However, a study in which participants continued training three times a week during one year showed a sustained antihypertensive effect. Thus, even though additional studies are needed, the available evidence is sufficiently strong to recommend dynamic exercise to hypertensive individuals whose physical condition is suitable.

All these results have been obtained in unmedicated hypertensive patients. An unexplored area is that of the effects of exercise in hypertensive patients who are already on drug therapy. Indeed, even when drug therapy is required, hypertensive patients live a normal life when hypertension is detected early enough. That is to say, many start jogging, attend physical fitness classes, or learn swimming at some point after their hypertension has been diagnosed and treated.

Just how this could affect the action of medication is not known at present and requires further study. It's also possible for some blood pressure lowering drugs to affect a person's ability to exercise. For example, beta-blockers slow the heart rate and make it more difficult for people to improve their tolerance of exercise. This does not mean that people who are on beta-blockers shouldn't exercise. It simply means that people on beta-blockers will have to work a little harder to achieve the same level of physical activity. (Beta-blockers are discussed in chapter 8.)

Practical recommendations for exercise. Exercise is not beneficial for everyone. Indeed, the recommendations of the Canadian Consensus Conference suggest that it may be of benefit only for those attempting to lose weight.

If you and your doctor feel that you should increase your exercise, here are some tips on how to get started. First, you must be willing to become more physically active in everyday life. This by no means implies that you should rush off to register for fitness classes right away! Rather, you should begin with more convenient measures. For instance, you could get off the bus one stop earlier and walk the remaining distance to your destination. Or you could use the stairs instead of the elevator, or get off the elevator one floor earlier. (We recommend that you start by walking downstairs for a few weeks before walking upstairs. This will impose less of a burden on your heart while improving the strength of your leg muscles.)

These are obvious suggestions. You can probably think of many other methods to increase routine exercise. With the tight schedules of modern life, you may have to make some minor concessions to change your exercise habits. For example, you'll have to leave earlier for work if you choose to walk. You may have to take ten minutes less for lunch if you take the stairs to and from the cafeteria instead of the elevator. If you aren't willing to sacrifice the time needed to make these changes, it's unlikely that you'll adhere to the demands of a fitness program that involves even more time and expense. On the other hand, if you find it rewarding to perform a certain physical activity without much discomfort (e.g., if walking for 30 minutes in the evening before supper becomes an enjoyable part of your day), then you probably are the type of person who could benefit further from a carefully supervised exercise program.

At this point, you could start looking for more specialized advice as to the type of exercise you need. To begin, tell your doctor about your more active lifestyle, then ask his advice. He might be able to refer you to an exercise physiologist who could assess your general fitness level and recommend an individualized training program for you. As your fitness level increases and as a significant antihypertensive effect of exercise becomes evident, your doctor may want to postpone drug treatment.

On the other hand, if you're already taking antihypertensive medication, the type or the dosage of drug might have to be changed. We emphasize that your doctor must be involved in such decisions. Do not try to replace medication with exercise! This might be the wrong decision. Such action may be appropriate only in the long term.

An exercise program must last longer than six weeks before significant effects can be seen. Up to 20 weeks are required to achieve maximal antihypertensive effect. Remember that your goal should be a general change in your lifestyle, from sedentary to more active. It isn't possible to achieve this overnight. Depending on your initial fitness level, it can take up to a year before you are ready to join a true training program. Be patient!

CONCLUSION

Some aspects of lifestyle, including excess weight and alcohol consumption, affect blood pressure. You can read about diet and weight in chapter 4, and we've talked about alcohol in detail. Regular exercise also appears to have an effect on blood pressure and is helpful with weight reduction. The evidence is not yet firm on the value of the relaxation/stress management method.

6

Drug Therapy — A General Approach

Martin Myers, M.D.

In this chapter, we'll briefly explain the various types of drugs used to treat high blood pressure. More information on them can be found in chapters 7–11.

RECENT HISTORY

In the past 50 years, few advances in medicine have surpassed the benefits achieved by the development of drugs for the treatment of high blood pressure. Before 1950, there was no effective way to lower blood pressure with or without medications. When a doctor made a diagnosis of high blood pressure, it was generally received with great despair since the outcome was often quite dismal. Indeed, patients with the most severe type of high blood pressure had less than a 10 percent chance of surviving the next 12 months.

Fortunately, medical research and the development of new drugs for the treatment of high blood pressure have almost completely reversed this gloomy outcome. Between 1950 and 1970, drug treatment of hypertension became increasingly widespread. Most of the attention during this period was directed toward patients with more severe high blood pressure because the drugs often caused troublesome side-effects and were appropriate only for those most likely to benefit. However, by the early 1970s, the availability of agents such as diuretics and beta-blockers made it possible to treat most hypertensives with a minimum of side-effects.

It was thus disappointing when surveys in the early 1970s indicated that less than a quarter of hypertensive patients were receiving adequate treatment, despite the availability of effective medication. Major efforts were undertaken to alert both patients and doctors to the importance of treating high blood pressure. By the mid-1980s, most hypertensives were being properly treated, and their blood pressure was under control.

DEVELOPMENT OF NEW DRUGS

During the past 20 years, many types of medication have become available for the treatment of high blood pressure. Before reaching the local pharmacy, these new drugs are tested extensively. Studies are done, first in animals and then in humans, to determine how well a drug lowers blood pressure and to make certain that it's free of serious adverse effects.

The results of these initial studies are carefully evaluated by both the pharmaceutical company developing the drug and by the Bureau of Drugs of the Health Protection Branch in Ottawa. This regulatory process is extremely demanding. It often takes years before a new drug reaches the patient, despite pressure from the drug company, doctors and the public to have potentially useful treatments approved for general use as quickly as possible.

The news media sometimes unknowingly promote new drugs when they report on promising new treatments. We must recognize that a new drug is not necessarily a better one with fewer side-effects. Unless you're having difficulty with the medication you currently take, there's no need to request treatment with a new drug even if a newspaper article or TV program suggests that it's a "wonder drug."

One final comment about new drugs: advances in the treatment of high blood pressure are made possible only because of the co-operation of patients like you. One reason we currently have so many safe drugs is that patients are willing to participate in carefully designed studies (refer to chapter 3). Without the patients' help, we'd still be in the same situation as 10 or 20 years ago when there were only a few drugs available that frequently caused side-effects. Better drugs are still needed! Many studies and many patients will be required if we're to improve upon what's currently available. If you're asked to participate in a study evaluating a new drug for the treatment of high blood pressure, please give it your serious consideration. You, your children or your neighbor may benefit from participation in this type of research.

TREATMENT GOALS

We know that lowering blood pressure to less than 140/90 mmHg will reduce complications. However, there is less certainty about the best blood pressure to aim for. In general, among individuals who are not on treatment, the lower the blood pressure the better. However, there is some evidence that lowering the blood pressure far below 140/90 mmHg may not give added benefit; indeed, it may run the risk of more adverse effects. At the moment, the goal is to lower blood pressure to less than 140/90 mmHg, with the understanding that going to very low levels with drugs may not give any added benefits.

LOWERING BLOOD PRESSURE

In patients with mild hypertension, the ideal approach is to reduce blood pressure without drugs. For example, an obese patient can lose weight, heavy users of alcohol can drink less, and everyone can consume less salt (sodium) in their diet. As explained in chapter 15, however, it's often difficult for people to follow these instructions. Even if followed, they'll often reduce the blood pressure by only a small amount in comparison with drug treatments. For patients with more than just a slight increase in blood pressure, and for those who find it difficult to stick with non-drug treatments, medication must be used.

In general, drugs reduce blood pressure by influencing mechanisms that are involved in the normal maintenance of blood pressure. Think of your heart as a pump and the blood vessels as hoses attached to that pump. We can use drugs to change the activity of the pump (the heart), or to change the resistance of the hoses (blood vessels) to the flow of blood. Using drugs, we can decrease the heart rate and the amount of blood pumped out of the heart to the body (for example, with beta-blockers), or we can reduce the resistance to blood flow (for example, with vasodilators).

DRUGS CURRENTLY AVAILABLE

Now we turn to the medications that are used to treat high blood pressure today. They've been grouped into five main categories to give you an overview. Details of each type of drug are in the chapters indicated.

Diuretics (water pills)

Diuretics increase the amount of sodium (salt) and water excreted by the kidneys as urine. This action reduces the volume of blood pumped by the heart with each beat. Diuretics may also decrease the sodium content of blood vessels, leading to reduced resistance to flow (see also chapter 7).

Inhibitors of the sympathetic nervous system

The sympathetic nervous system is part of the autonomic nervous system described in chapter 1. Through it, the brain sends signals that act on the heart and the blood vessels. The sympathetic nervous system works via two hormones (noradrenaline and adrenaline) that stimulate receptors on the walls of some cells of the body. There are two main types of receptors, alpha and beta. Stimulation of the alpha-receptors causes constriction (narrowing) of the blood vessels, and stimulation of the beta-receptors causes the heart to pump harder. Because stimulation of either alpha- or beta-receptors can raise blood pressure, drugs that block these receptors thus lower the blood pressure. Drugs that inhibit the sympathetic nervous system include alpha-blockers, beta-blockers, and drugs that work directly in the brain (centrally acting drugs) to reduce the stimulating effects of the sympathetic nervous system (see also chapter 8).

Angiotensin-converting enzyme (ACE) inhibitors

These drugs block the effects of the hormone renin, which is released from the kidney. Renin normally acts to produce other hormones (angiotensins) that constrict arteries. By blocking the actions of renin, ACE inhibitors relax arteries and lower the resistance to blood flow (see also chapter 9).

Calcium antagonists

These drugs inhibit the entry of calcium into muscle cells in the heart and in the walls of arteries. Because calcium is needed for muscle contraction, these drugs decrease the heart's power of contraction and output of blood. They also act as vasodilators (see below) to reduce the resistance of blood flow in the arteries (see also chapter 10).

Vasodilators

Vasodilators relax the muscle in the walls of arteries. This action widens these blood vessels and thus decreases the resistance to blood flow (see also chapter 11).

THE IDEAL DRUG

The ideal drug for hypertension would reduce blood pressure without causing any adverse effects. It would be inexpensive, would require infrequent administration, and would eliminate all the complications of high blood pressure. It would also be compatible with other drugs and not be affected by other diseases or medical conditions. As you might expect, we haven't yet achieved perfection. Fortunately, we do have a variety of drugs available that lower blood pressure effectively and have many of these other positive attributes.

CANADIAN RECOMMENDATIONS FOR DRUG TREATMENT

The Canadian Hypertension Society recently held a Consensus Conference to develop recommendations on the drug treatment of hypertension. In its discussions, the Conference used the "ideal" drug as a standard by which to judge currently available medications.

Selecting the drug with the most favorable characteristics isn't simple. For example, a new drug may lower blood pressure effectively and seem to be comparatively free of side-effects. It's usually more expensive, however, because it costs a great deal to produce and test a new drug. In addition, the new drug won't have been around long enough for us to know if it has any long-term adverse effects or if it actually reduces the complications of hypertension over a five- to ten-year period. Thus, an older, less-expensive and better-known medication has its attractions.

Any recommendations on the drug treatment of high blood pressure must take into account what we know about each drug and what has yet to be discovered, particularly with the newer agents.

TREATMENT OF PATIENTS WITH UNCOMPLICATED HIGH BLOOD PRESSURE

Diuretics or beta-blockers are recommended as the first choice in treating most hypertensive patients who don't have complications or other conditions that might influence the selection of appropriate therapy. Current practice is to recommend lower doses of diuretics (e.g., hydrochlorothiazide 25–50 mg per day). This is because we now know that the higher doses used previously weren't necessary to lower blood pressure. These unnecessarily high doses were the main reason many patients experienced adverse effects such as low potassium in the blood (see chapter 7 for details).

A beta-blocker or diuretic can be expected to produce normal blood pressure in about two-thirds of patients with mild or moderate hypertension. Sometimes, however, the blood pressure is not lowered enough with the first medication. Rather than adding a second drug at this point, your doctor may try an alternate medication on its own; for example, if a beta-blocker has not reduced the blood pressure enough, it could be replaced with a diuretic.

If the blood pressure isn't brought down to normal with the diuretic or beta-blocker alone, there are several options, as outlined in Figure 1. For instance, the beta-blocker and diuretic can be combined in small doses. Alternatively, when the beta-blocker and diuretic have each been tried alone and have failed to normalize the blood pressure, another agent such as an ACE inhibitor, calcium antagonist or centrally acting drug (in order of preference) may be prescribed. The aim is to reduce the blood pressure to normal while using only one medication. These agents may also be used if the combination of beta-blocker and diuretic has not produced satisfactory results.

Some patients with more severe high blood pressure, or those whose blood pressure is somewhat resistant to treatment, may require other combinations of drugs. Commonly used combinations include a diuretic with an ACE inhibitor, a centrally acting drug or an alpha-blocker. Alternatively, a beta-blocker can be given with a calcium antagonist, a vasodilator or an alpha-blocker. If the use of two drugs doesn't produce a normal blood pressure, then three or more agents may be required. Fortunately, this situation arises in less than 10 percent of patients with high blood pressure.

If there are no complicating factors influencing the choice of therapy, the doctor can follow the general approach outlined above. When the high blood pressure is more difficult to control, it's often necessary to try several different combinations. The goal is to find one or more medications that lower blood pressure adequately with few or no side-effects at a reasonable cost and a minimum number of tablets per day.

Just because your doctor doesn't initially prescribe the

right drug or combination of drugs doesn't necessarily mean that he isn't treating you properly. For reasons that are usually unknown, some patients will respond better to one type of medicine than another. It sometimes takes several attempts before the best drug(s) are matched to the patient.

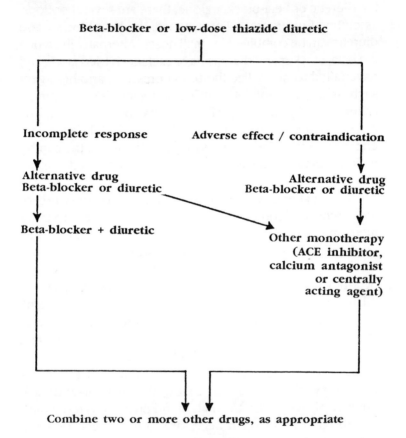

Figure 1: Usual approach to prescribing drugs for uncomplicated hypertension.

(Originally published in *Canadian Medical Association Journal,* Vol.140, May 15, 1989.)

TREATMENT OF HIGH BLOOD PRESSURE IN THE PRESENCE OF OTHER DISORDERS

A doctor may prefer a particular drug for treating hypertension because a patient has another condition that might also benefit from the same medicine. On the other hand, it may not be possible to prescribe certain drugs if a patient has another medical condition that would be adversely affected by the treatment. To select the most appropriate blood pressure drug, the doctor will check the patient (as described in chapter 2) for the presence of illnesses such as heart disease, stroke, diabetes, high cholesterol, kidney disease, asthma and gout.

Heart disease

Patients with high blood pressure *and* coronary artery disease (i.e., those who have had a heart attack or who suffer from angina) are often prescribed beta-blockers or calcium antagonists. These drugs are beneficial in that they treat both the hypertension and the heart disease.

Diuretics and ACE inhibitors are often used to treat patients who have congestive heart failure, which usually involves damage to the heart muscle and an impaired pumping action of the heart. If a patient also has high blood pressure, then a diuretic and/or ACE inhibitor may be used to benefit both conditions. Some drugs may be harmful if heart failure is a major concern. In these instances, beta-blockers and calcium antagonists should be avoided.

Diabetes

Special considerations may be necessary for patients who have both diabetes and high blood pressure. If a diabetic patient is not taking insulin, diuretics are generally avoided because they often increase the blood sugar and may make control of the diabetes more difficult. However, if a patient is using insulin, any effect of the diuretic on blood sugar is of less importance because changes in the blood sugar can be controlled simply by altering the dose of insulin.

Further information on the treatment of high blood pressure in diabetics can be found in chapter 13.

High cholesterol

Some of the best and most widely used drugs for treating high blood pressure can cause an increase in cholesterol and other fatty substances (triglycerides) in the body. For example, we know that taking high doses of a diuretic for a couple of months can increase blood cholesterol levels by about five percent; however, we don't know if this effect persists with long-term use. Also, the lower doses of diuretics that are currently recommended have less of an effect on cholesterol and may not cause much increase in most patients. Some beta-blockers also cause small increases in fatty substances in the blood, especially triglycerides. Other drugs, such as alpha-blockers, ACE inhibitors, calcium antagonists and centrally acting drugs, do not increase cholesterol or triglyceride levels.

If cholesterol is a special concern, why would your doctor prescribe a beta-blocker or diuretic that might increase it? The answer is that we have to consider the pros and cons of each medication. Diuretics and beta-blockers effectively lower blood pressure, have been shown to reduce death, are inexpensive and have adverse effects that are well known because these drugs have been around for so long. Most of the newer drugs that have no effect on cholesterol have not yet been shown to reduce death, and they are comparatively expensive.

The Canadian Hypertension Society proposed a compromise: if cholesterol or triglycerides are of special concern (for example, in a patient with already high levels), the doctor should perform regular blood tests to monitor levels of cholesterol and triglycerides after starting a medication that might increase these levels. Any sign of worsening in a patient's cholesterol or triglyceride levels should lead to consideration of an alternate medication. For patients with normal cholesterol levels, the usual treatment for high blood pressure is appropriate.

Asthma

Beta-blockers should not be used in patients who have had asthma (wheezy breathing not necessarily associated with a respiratory infection). These drugs tend to make breathing more difficult.

Gout

Diuretics can increase the amount of uric acid in the blood. Increased amounts of this substance can accumulate in the body, causing gout (severe joint inflammation and pain). Gout can usually be treated effectively with other medication. If the diuretic was the cause of the gout, stopping the diuretic will generally prevent further attacks.

Special circumstances

Pregnant women may develop high blood pressure, but this often clears up with bed rest. Drug therapy is sometimes required. Caution with drug treatment in pregnancy is extremely important, and only a few compounds are recommended: methyldopa, hydralazine and beta-blockers. In special circumstances, other drugs may be used with care if they are not known to be harmful for the mother or fetus and the blood pressure can't be controlled otherwise. Further details are provided in chapter 14.

In the elderly, diuretics are generally preferred over beta-blockers because they seem to be somewhat more effective. We tend to use smaller doses of most drugs in older patients and take special care to avoid inducing any side-effects. More information is given in chapter 12.

Black patients may respond particularly well to diuretics and so one of these drugs is often prescribed first. Otherwise, treatment is the same as outlined above.

SIDE-EFFECTS OF BLOOD PRESSURE-LOWERING DRUGS

Nearly all drugs currently used to treat high blood pressure are well tolerated. No drug, however, is totally without adverse effects. Most side-effects are harmless and readily tolerated by patients. If a side-effect (e.g., nausea, headache, cough, flushing, constipation) is troublesome, the doctor will usually prescribe another drug. If it's extremely important to use a particular drug, then the side-effect may be treated in a specific way (e.g., a laxative for constipation). With some drugs, periodic blood tests or electrocardiograms are needed to monitor for possible adverse effects that may not be noticed by the patient.

Some people experience discomfort with virtually every drug they receive. Often this isn't due to the drug itself but to the person's dislike of being on medication. This presents a difficult problem for both the patient and the doctor. Some ways to deal with it are discussed in chapter 15. Even with this problem, it's important to remember that blood pressure lowering treatments reduce the complications of high blood pressure and that they can work only if taken regularly!

If you feel that a drug is bothersome, tell your doctor. *Don't* stop taking it on your own. Some drugs may cause problems if they are stopped suddenly. Only your doctor knows the best way of changing your medication.

7

Diuretics

S. G. Carruthers, M.D. and C. R. Dean, M.D.

Diuretics (water pills) lower blood pressure by reducing the amount of water and salt in the body and relaxing the blood vessels. A low dose of a thiazide diuretic is a fairly common way of starting to treat mild or moderate hypertension. Together with beta-blockers (discussed in chapters 6 and 8), they're recommended as initial (starting) treatment, and are convenient because they're taken once a day. Diuretics are also useful for people who have heart failure.

HOW DIURETICS WORK

A diuretic increases the amount of salt and water that the kidneys remove from the body. The salt is sodium chloride — just like regular table salt. You may notice that, with the first few doses of a diuretic, you make more urine than usual. The loss of this extra fluid can result in a small decrease in body weight of about one-half to two kilograms (1–4 pounds). The body acts very quickly to protect itself against the loss of too much water and salt, which could be harmful. After a few days there will be a new balance, with a little less water and salt in the body. The diuretic is still working, but you will no longer be aware of passing more urine than usual.

Your blood pressure will gradually decrease because there is a smaller volume of fluid in your circulation than before the diuretic was started. Because there is a smaller volume, there is less blood reaching the heart during each beat. In addition, the amount of salt in the walls of the blood vessels decreases and causes them to dilate (or open up). This causes less resistance for the heart to pump against and helps the fall in blood pressure.

In older patients, diuretics tend to lower blood pressure quite effectively. Younger patients' bodies tend to adjust well to the effects of diuretics, however, and their blood pressure may remain the same or increase slightly. These drugs are favored, therefore, in older people and are used less often in younger individuals, where they may not work as well.

TYPES OF DIURETICS

There are four main groups of diuretics: thiazides or thiazide-like diuretics; potassium-sparing diuretics; combination diuretics; and loop diuretics. Table 1 gives more details and examples of each group. Only commonly used diuretics have been mentioned. All drugs have both brand (trade) name(s) and a chemical (generic) name. Ask your doctor or pharmacist for the chemical name if you're in doubt as to what kind of drug you're getting, because different companies make similar drugs under different brand names. Newer drugs usually have just one brand name and one chemical name. Drugs that have been on the market for several years sometimes have two or more brand names. This is because they are manufactured by different companies. However, they still have only one chemical name.

Table 1: Commonly Prescribed Diuretics

Class	Chemical name	Brand name	Usual daily dose (mg)
Thiazide-like	chlorthalidone	Hygroton	12.5 - 25
		Uridon	12.5 - 25
	hydrochlorothiazide	Hydro-diuril	25 - 50
		Esidrex	25 - 50
	indapamide	Lozide	2.5
Potassium-sparing	amiloride	Midamor	*
	spironolactone	Aldactone	25 - 100
	triamterene	Dyrenium	*
Combination	hydrochlorothiazide		
	+ amiloride	Moduret	1 - 2 tablets
	+ spironolactone	Aldactazide	1 - 2 tablets
	+ triamterene	Dyazide	1 - 2 tablets
Loop	furosemide	Lasix	20 - 80

* These medications are rarely used alone.

Thiazide diuretics

The thiazide or thiazide-like diuretics are often known as thiazides for short. Their effect is usually mild, comes on gradually, and lasts a relatively long time. You may not notice any difference in the amount of urine you produce when you start taking them; just the same, most people prefer to take them in the morning to avoid having to get up in the middle of the night. This is the type of diuretic that's most often used in the treatment of mild to moderate hypertension. The thiazides are also commonly used in more severe hypertension. In this case they're given in combination with one or more of the other medicines described in this book such as beta-blockers or ACE inhibitors.

Potassium-sparing diuretics

Potassium is an important mineral for the functioning of all body tissues. Thiazide and loop diuretics sometimes cause low potassium, which can lead to weakness or tiredness of the muscles and heart trouble. Potassium-sparing diuretics act on the kidneys in a different way from thiazides or loop diuretics, so that potassium loss is small. Sometimes these medications actually lead to an increase of potassium in the blood and tissues. They tend to be rather weak at lowering blood pressure, however, so they're not often used by themselves. Spironolactone is the exception, being used in some forms of high blood pressure that are associated with too great a loss of potassium or a lot of salt being held in the body. In patients with poor kidneys and in patients who are taking other medications that keep potassium in the body, there's a risk that the potassium level can increase too much. If this is the case, your doctor might measure the level of potassium in your blood by a simple test.

Combination diuretics

These drugs are mixtures of a thiazide and one of the potassium-sparing medicines. They generally keep the blood level of potassium normal. However, they tend to be more expensive and usually cause only a little more lowering of blood pressure than the thiazides alone.

Loop diuretics

In contrast to the thiazides, loop diuretics act very quickly. They can cause a large loss of fluid over a short time. Shortly after taking these pills, most people have to pass urine several times. Therefore, it's not a good idea to take such a tablet just before driving the car or going to the supermarket! Most people prefer taking this type of diuretic shortly after they get up in the morning so the effects have worn off before they go out. If you have an appointment in the morning, you may choose to delay taking the medicine until you get home again.

In the hours after this type of diuretic has stopped working, the body compensates for the salt and water losses by holding on to fluid, so there is very little urine output for a while. Because of their large effect on urine output and the short duration of this effect, loop diuretics are usually prescribed for the treatment of high blood pressure only when there are other complications. They're very useful, however, in patients who have heart failure. They're also useful in patients who have a decrease in kidney function. Sometimes they're used, in combination with other medications, in the treatment of severe hypertension.

SIDE-EFFECTS OF DIURETICS

Most people do not experience any bad side-effects from using diuretics. However, a thiazide diuretic can cause several chemical changes in the body that may lead to the following problems.

Increase in blood sugar

Diuretics increase blood sugar slightly in most people. Generally, this is not a problem, but in people with a tendency to develop diabetes, this increase in blood sugar may be enough to bring out the symptoms of diabetes. Any increase in thirst or passing larger amounts of urine after you have been taking the diuretic for a few weeks should be discussed with your doctor. In patients with diabetes controlled by diet alone or by diet plus pills, diuretics might make diabetes worse. Obviously, if at all possible, the use of diuretics in such patients will be avoided.

Decrease in blood potassium (hypokalemia)

Diuretics cause the loss not only of salt and water but also of other chemicals in the body (known as *electrolytes*) such as potassium. If blood potassium decreases too much, your muscles will not function as well and you may feel tired. In patients with heart trouble, particularly in those using the heart drug digoxin, the heart muscle is very sensitive to a low level of blood potassium and may beat irregularly.

Very few otherwise healthy people experience any side-effects because the blood potassium level is too low. If this does happen, it can be treated easily. This is done by giving extra potassium by mouth or by switching to a potassium-sparing diuretic. A small fall in potassium is not a serious matter unless you have heart disease and are on digoxin. If your potassium level falls a lot while you are on a small dose of thiazide, your doctor might want to check how your kidneys are working. He may decide to check the blood supply to the kidneys, and he may also want to check how the adrenal glands, which control salt and water (refer to chapters 1 and 2), are working.

Increase in blood uric acid

Uric acid is a chemical produced by the body and excreted in the urine. It causes gout if too much stays in the body. In this disease, crystals of uric acid make the lining of a joint inflamed and sore. It typically shows up as a red, tender, painful big toe, but other joints can also be affected. Diuretics sometimes cause an increase in uric acid and can start an attack of gout in those who have a tendency to it. Fortunately, most people are not inclined that way. If the uric acid level in your blood goes up a little, your doctor likely won't treat it. It usually doesn't lead to any harm. If you do have an acute attack of gout, it may be necessary to stop your diuretic. Sometimes other medicines, such as allopurinol, are used to help cut down the amount of uric acid that your body makes.

Increase in blood cholesterol

Cholesterol is a fatty material that can be found in the blood. It's necessary for making some very important hormones and for making membranes that surround body cells. If the amount of cholesterol in the blood becomes too great, there's an increased chance of heart attack. Unfortunately, the level of cholesterol can be increased by diuretics. It's recommended that the blood cholesterol level be checked before medication is started. It might also be checked again after the treatment has been given for several months. If your doctor finds that your cholesterol level is too high, you may have to make some changes in your diet or try another treatment for the high blood pressure.

Other problems

Besides these chemical changes, some people may notice dizziness upon standing. Sometimes men suffer from impotence, or a decrease in sexual function, after taking diuretics for a while. Occasionally, diuretics may cause too much fluid loss or dehydration. This can occur when the doses of the diuretics are too high. Dehydration may also occur in people who don't drink enough water and in people who sweat a lot in very hot weather. It may also occur in people with a bad attack of diarrhea. If you think that you have any of these problems and may be dehydrated, you should see your doctor.

PREVENTING SIDE-EFFECTS

What can we do about these side-effects? The most important prevention is to use low doses. In recent years we've learned that low doses of thiazides work as well as larger doses for lowering blood pressure. With low doses, the chance of any side-effect is much less. For example, doctors now use as little as 12.5 mg daily of chlorthalidone or hydrochlorothiazide, instead of up to 100 mg a day as we once prescribed several years ago. We see hardly any side-effects at these low doses. If side-effects still occur, the best approach is to stop the diuretic and try another medication to lower the blood pressure.

Sometimes, however, a patient needs a diuretic. For example, if someone has high blood pressure and a heart problem, it may be necessary to relieve the heart by lowering the amount of fluid in the body. In such cases we may have to accept a side effect and treat it.

In heart patients, the decrease in blood potassium is a side effect that we don't want. One way to prevent this is to eat foods rich in potassium (most fresh fruits and vegetables, particularly bananas, oranges and potatoes), or to take potassium tablets. However, potassium tablets are expensive and don't always prevent a decrease in blood potassium. Many tablets may be necessary to get enough potassium into the body. A better and simpler way is to combine the regular diuretic with a potassium-sparing one (see "combination tablets" in table 1). Most healthy persons whose only problem is high blood pressure and who use low doses of a diuretic don't need these combination diuretics or additional potassium tablets. If you're concerned about low blood potassium, it's better to eat more fresh fruits and vegetables. Refer to chapter 4 for more information.

Another good way to reduce the chance of your potassium level getting too low is to cut down on the amount of salt in your diet. This also helps the diuretic do its job of lowering blood pressure.

Although low doses of thiazide diuretics make the chance of these chemical changes much lower, the doctor will want to do blood tests from time to time to make sure that no important changes occur after you start these pills. This is one of the disadvantages of the diuretics and is why some doctors and patients don't like using them. The extra lab tests do add to the cost, but diuretics are still very inexpensive unless many lab tests are done.

8

Drugs and the Sympathetic Nervous System

Jack Onrot, M.D., Tom Wilson, M.D., and Merne Dubois, R.N.

In this chapter we'll discuss drugs that affect the sympathetic nervous system: alpha- and beta-blockers, centrally acting agents (clonidine and methyldopa) and the older drugs such as reserpine and guanethidine.

As explained in chapter 1, the involuntary (or *autonomic*) nervous system plays an important role in the control of blood pressure. The autonomic nervous system is divided into two major parts, the parasympathetic and the sympathetic nervous systems. It's the sympathetic nervous system that, when activated, raises blood pressure. This is the same system that produces the well-known fight-or-flight response, which occurs when a person is in a threatening situation. By blocking the activity of this system, certain drugs can lower blood pressure.

The sympathetic nervous system is controlled by the brain stem, the lowest part of the brain, located just above the spinal cord. Sympathetic nerve impulses travel from the brain stem down the spinal cord, and they transfer their information to nerve fibres that travel to the heart, blood vessels and other important tissues, as shown in figure 1.

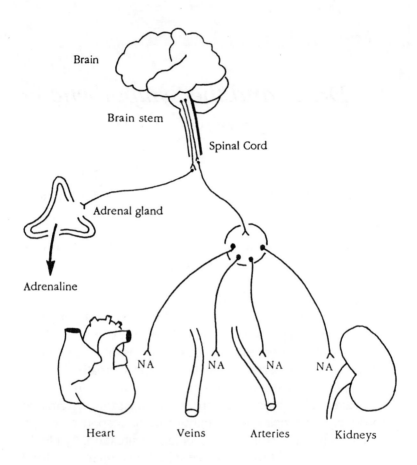

Figure 1: The autonomic nervous system.

(Nerve impulses travel from the brain stem down the spinal cord to the nerves, the heart, the blood vessels, and other tissues.)

* NA = noradrenaline

When a sympathetic nerve is stimulated, a chemical (noradrenaline) is released from the nerve ending. The noradrenaline binds to its own receptors located on target tissues such as the heart and blood vessels. There are two types of receptors for noradrenaline, called alpha and beta. Beta-1-receptors in the heart, when activated by noradrenaline, cause the heart to beat faster and more strongly (thus raising blood pressure). Alpha-receptors on the blood vessels cause them to narrow, raising blood pressure. Beta-2-receptors on blood vessels cause them to open up. Adrenaline, from the adrenal gland, circulates in the blood and also activates these receptors (this is outlined in figure 2). Blocking alpha- and beta-1-receptors is one way of opposing sympathetic nervous system activity and lowering blood pressure.

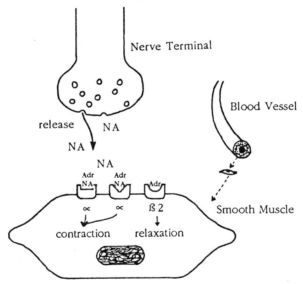

Figure 2: Sympathetic nerve terminal at a blood vessel.

(When a nerve impulse reaches this terminal, noradrenaline (NA) is released. It attaches to receptors and causes the blood vessels to contract. Adrenaline (Adr) circulates in the blood stream. It stimulates beta-receptors (B_2), which can relax the blood vessels.)

BETA-BLOCKERS

Beta-blockers block the action of noradrenaline and adrenaline at beta-receptors located in specific target tissues in the body. Because beta-receptors, when stimulated, increase the force of contraction of the heart and the heart rate, beta-blockers can oppose these actions and reduce blood pressure. Beta-receptors also affect renin secretion by the kidney to raise blood pressure (for details, refer to chapters 1 and 9), and so beta-blockers also oppose this action.

Beta-blockers tend to be more effective in younger patients and less effective in the over-65 age group. They're also less effective in black patients. Beta-blockers are useful for people in whom high sympathetic nervous system activity is suspected, such as very anxious patients or patients who have relatively high heart rates. Beta-blockers are often used in many other medical conditions, and when these conditions co-exist with hypertension, it's clearly an advantage to use one drug to treat two problems. On the other hand, there are also conditions for which beta-blockers may be harmful, and it's best to use other medications if possible.

Table 1 gives a brief list of conditions that will benefit or suffer from the use of beta-blockers. Note that these are guidelines only. Your doctor will take other factors into account in making the decision about whether a beta-blocker should be prescribed. The "Avoid if" column is a reasonably full list of potential side-effects of beta-blockers.

Beta-receptors in the heart differ somewhat from those located elsewhere. *Selective* beta-blockers such as atenolol, metoprolol and acebutolol are so named because they block beta-1-receptors in the heart more than beta-2-receptors elsewhere. It's sometimes advantageous to avoid blocking non-cardiac beta-2-receptors because they can open up blood vessels and air tubes (*bronchi*) to the lung. Blocking this beta-2 "opening-up" action with beta-blockers might cause asthma or reduced circulation to fingers and legs. In the case of asthma, none of the beta-blockers is safe; beta-blockers should be avoided.

Table 1: Some Factors Influencing Choice of Beta-blockers

Choose if	Avoid if
Previous heart attack	asthma/emphysema
Angina	Raynaud's phenomenon
Rapid heart rhythms	peripheral artery blockage
	(claudication)
Migraines	diabetes
Tremor	slow heart rhythms
Anxiety	heart failure
Overactive thyroid	depression
Glaucoma	impotence
Aneurysm of aorta	elevated cholesterol/triglycerides
	chronic fatigue
	sleep disturbances
	exercise intolerance

Beta-blockers may have side-effects. Besides aggravating asthma and reducing blood circulation on occasion, they can also cause fatigue and decreased ability to exercise. Less often, they may worsen heart failure. They may also cause or worsen depression, disturb sleep and interfere with sexual function. Fortunately, these side-effects are not common and disappear when the drug is stopped.

Some beta-blockers actually exert a mild stimulant effect on beta-receptors. Examples of these agents are acebutolol, pindolol, and oxprenolol. These drugs are useful in treating patients who have low heart rates. They also may have advantages over other beta-blockers in the treatment of hypertensive patients with high cholesterol since this group of beta-blockers does not increase cholesterol.

Certain beta-blockers dissolve better in water than in fat (i.e., they're *water-soluble*) whereas other beta-blockers dissolve better in fat than water (i.e., they're *lipid-soluble*). Because the barrier separating the brain's circulation from the body's circulation is made of lipids, lipid-soluble beta-blockers tend to enter the brain more easily. Certain beta-blocker side-effects are due to the entry of the drug into the brain. They include nightmares, depression, fatigue and impotence. These problems occur less often with the water-soluble beta-blockers, which include nadolol, atenolol, and acebutolol.

A unique beta-blocker, labetalol, also has mild alpha-blocking activity, which provides an additional blood pressure-lowering effect. (For more information, see the next section on alpha-blockers.)

The various beta-blockers, their brand names, usual dosages and types of action are listed in table 2.

Table 2: Characteristics of Beta-blockers

Chemical name	Brand name	Usual daily dosage (mg)	Beta-1 selective	Water-soluble	ISA*
Acebutolol	Monitan Sectral	200–800	+	+	+
Atenolol	Tenormin	25–100	+	+	-
Labetalol	Trandate	200–800	-	-	-
Metoprolol	Betaloc Lopresor	25–200	+	-	-
Nadolol	Corgard	20–80	-	+	-
Oxprenolol	Trasicor	60–320	-	-	+
Pindolol	Visken	5–30	-	-	+
Propranolol	Inderal	40–320	-	-	-
Timolol	Blocadren	5–40	-	-	-

* intrinsic sympathomimetic activity (mild stimulant effect)
+ drug has this property
- drug does not have this property

ALPHA-BLOCKERS

The two alpha-blockers, prazosin and terazosin, block the action of noradrenaline and adrenaline at alpha-receptors on blood vessels. Because noradrenaline and adrenaline narrow blood vessels, blocking their action will relax blood vessels and lower blood pressure.

Alpha-blockers can be used alone for hypertension, but they're usually used in combination with other drugs. They're often most effective when first used, losing some degree of effectiveness with prolonged use. Combining these agents with other drugs such as diuretics can prevent, or at least reduce, this gradual loss of effectiveness.

Alpha-blockers have one advantage over all other anti-hypertensive agents in that they actually lower cholesterol in the blood. Although this effect is moderate, it may be important in patients with already elevated cholesterol levels. Most of the other drugs have no effect on cholesterol, but certain classes may raise cholesterol (for example, diuretics in high doses and non-selective beta-blockers).

A small percentage of patients will have a profound fall in blood pressure and may even faint after the first dose of an alpha-blocker or after an increase in dose. This is known as the *first-dose effect.* Although this effect is rare, it can be minimized by giving a very small initial dose (0.5 mg) and starting it at bedtime, when the patient is unlikely to be getting up during the next two or three hours. It should be emphasized that this first-dose effect is encountered only when taking the first pill or when dosage is increased. Other side effects sometimes occur, including fatigue, light-headedness, headaches and upset stomach.

DRUGS THAT WORK IN THE BRAIN
(centrally acting drugs)

These drugs, such as methyldopa and clonidine, reduce the flow of messages from the brain through sympathetic nerves. This lowers the blood pressure.

These drugs are useful because they don't have any adverse effects on lipids or electrolytes (such as potassium) in the blood. Because they act in the brain, the most commonly encountered side-effects are fatigue, sedation, or even confusion. These drugs may also cause impotence in men, reduction of libido (sex drive) in women, dry mouth, and stuffy nose. Because the sympathetic nervous system is essential for maintaining blood pressure when we stand up, these agents can also be associated with upright blood pressures that are too low. This produces light-headedness or even fainting. Methyldopa has a slow and long-acting effect. In contrast, clonidine acts quickly and also disappears quickly. Stopping clonidine suddenly can result in a withdrawal syndrome, with rapid heartbeat, anxiety, and high blood pressure. Gradual withdrawal is therefore advisable if the drug must be stopped.

DRUGS THAT ACT ON SYMPATHETIC NERVE ENDINGS

Two drugs — guanethidine and reserpine — act on sympathetic nerve endings. Guanethidine prevents the release of noradrenaline by sympathetic nerves. Its side-effects are similar to those of the centrally acting agents but are much more commonly encountered. Guanethidine, because of its side-effects, is seldom used.

Reserpine depletes nerves of noradrenaline. It's one of the oldest known anti-hypertensive drugs but fell out of favor because of its tendency to cause depression. However, depression can be avoided by using low doses. Other side-effects are similar to those of other centrally acting agents. Some doctors favor the use of reserpine in selected patients because it has no adverse effects on lipids or electrolytes; it can also be given once a day, is often quite effective in small doses and is quite inexpensive.

Table 3 lists drugs (other than beta-blockers) that act on the sympathetic nervous system.

Table 3: Other Agents that Affect Sympathetic Activity

Chemical name	Brand name	Usual daily dosage (mg)	Type
Clonidine	Catapres	0.1 – 1.2	central agent
Methyldopa	Aldomet	250 – 2,000	central agent
Prazosin	Minipress	1.0 – 20	alpha-blocker
Reserpine	Serpasil	0.05 – 0.5	noradrenaline depletor
Terazosin	Hytrin	1.0 – 20	alpha-blocker

CONCLUSION

All the drugs described in this chapter share the common characteristic of reducing, in one way or another, nervous system activity. The drugs that work outside the brain (beta- and alpha-blockers) have fewer side-effects than centrally acting drugs and thus are often preferred by patients and their doctors. Nevertheless, centrally acting drugs are effective in lowering blood pressure and are often well tolerated by patients.

9

ACE Inhibitors

Louise F. Roy, M.D. and Frans H. H. Leenen, M.D., Ph.D.

ACE inhibitor is a short name for *angiotensin-converting-enzyme inhibitor* (it's easy to see why the name was shortened to ACE!). ACE inhibitors include several drugs that lower blood pressure by the same mechanism. Drugs in this class that are available in Canada are captopril (brand name Capoten) and enalapril (Vasotec).

HOW ACE INHIBITORS WORK

As described in chapters 1 and 2, the renin-angiotensin system helps in the regulation of normal blood pressure. In hypertension, the system may work at a level that's too high, raising the blood pressure above normal. The renin-angiotensin system is shown in figure 1.

The first step in this system is renin, a hormone produced by the kidneys. Renin is an enzyme that transforms a protein (angiotensinogen) into a smaller molecule, angiotensin I. Angiotensin I is transformed into angiotensin II by another enzyme — angiotensin-converting enzyme (ACE). Angiotensin II is a very potent hormone that narrows blood vessels. This increases the resistance of the vessels to blood flow and thus increases the blood pressure.

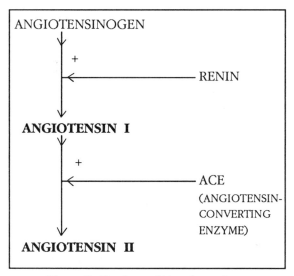

Figure 1: Renin-angiotensin system.

ACE inhibitors decrease the effect of the angiotensin-converting enzyme. The result is easy to predict: decreased production of angiotensin II. Figure 2 shows how, in the presence of ACE inhibitors, the quantity of angiotensin II in the blood will decrease, and thus so will blood pressure and the resistance of blood vessels. ACE inhibitors don't change heart rate or heart function. However, because they decrease vessel resistance and blood pressure, they decrease the amount of work that the heart has to perform. This improves heart activity in patients with heart failure.

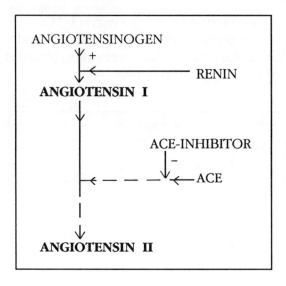

Figure 2: Renin-angiotensin system with ACE inhibitors.

At the moment there are two ACE inhibitors available in Canada; table 1 shows some of their characteristics. Another ACE inhibitor, lisinopril, is soon to be approved in Canada.

Table 1: ACE Inhibitors

Chemical name	Captopril	Enalapril
Brand name	Capoten	Vasotec
Starting dose	6.25–25 mg	2.5–5 mg
Average daily dose	25–100 mg	5–20 mg
Frequency of administration	2–4 times/day	1–2 times/day

WHEN ACE INHIBITORS ARE USED

ACE inhibitors may be used alone or in combination with other anti-hypertensive drugs. ACE inhibitors aren't equally effective in all patients. For example, black people respond to them less than white people. On the other hand, in patients taking diuretics (water pills), or on salt-restricted diets, ACE inhibitors are efficient blood pressure-lowering drugs. This is because the renin-angiotensin system is more active in these situations.

Patients suffering from heart failure, whether or not they have high blood pressure, often have increased activity of the renin-angiotensin system. ACE inhibitors may improve their symptoms of heart failure and improve their quality of life. Overall, ACE inhibitors are very effective for these patients. Large decreases of blood pressure may occur, however, so it's usual to start these patients on low doses.

Diabetics sometimes develop kidney disease. ACE inhibitors seem to be more effective than other blood pressure-lowering drugs in reducing kidney damage. However, they should not be used when certain other kidney diseases are present (see below).

Hypertension is sometimes caused by a narrowing of an artery that provides blood to one of the kidneys. In this case, ACE inhibitors also effectively lower blood pressure, particularly when used with a diuretic (refer to chapter 7).

WHEN ACE INHIBITORS ARE AVOIDED

The renin-angiotensin system plays an important role in the function of the kidneys. Because they inhibit the renin-angiotensin system, ACE inhibitors can impair the function of the kidneys. For this reason when the arteries to *both* kidneys are narrowed, ACE inhibitors should not be used. Fortunately, if ACE inhibitors are used in this case, the kidney function usually returns to its previous level when the drug is stopped.

Some patients may retain potassium because of a decrease in its excretion by the kidneys. This occurs most often when kidney function is poor. ACE inhibitors can aggravate this situation and should not be used in these patients.

Some drugs should not be used together with ACE inhibitors or must be used very carefully. These include potassium supplements, anti-inflammatory drugs (used in arthritis), and diuretics that cause potassium retention.

SIDE-EFFECTS OF ACE INHIBITORS

As mentioned earlier, ACE inhibitors may decrease kidney function, cause potassium accumulation, and produce large decreases in blood pressure in some patients. Fortunately, these effects are reversible and once the drug is discontinued, organ and body functions will revert to previous levels.

A dry cough may occur in a small percentage of patients; this is more common if lung disease is already present. Skin rashes occur in two to four percent of patients within the first two or three months. Taste disturbances occur in one or two percent of patients: some people experience a decrease in taste or a metallic-sour taste. Very rarely, the number of white blood cells may decrease.

Another rare occurrence, which may happen in the first month, is *angioedema*, or swelling of the mouth, lips and throat. **This is a dangerous side-effect: at the first sign, call a doctor immediately!**

All these side-effects are reversible and will disappear if the drug is stopped soon enough.

ACE inhibitors should not be used during pregnancy, as cases of malformed babies have been reported.

10

Calcium Antagonists

Louise F. Roy, M.D. and Frans H. H. Leenen, M.D., Ph.D.

Calcium antagonists, also known as calcium channel-blockers, are a class of drugs that work by interfering with the entry of calcium into cells. The calcium antagonists that are currently available for prescription in Canada are nifedipine (Adalat), diltiazem (Cardizem) and verapamil (Isoptin). There are several new calcium antagonists that may soon be available; their chemical names are felodipine, isradipine, nicardipine, nimodipine, nisoldipine and nitrendipine.

HOW CALCIUM ANTAGONISTS WORK

Calcium plays many roles inside the cells of the body. In blood vessel walls, calcium influences muscle cell contraction. To do so, it has to enter these cells through tiny channels in the cell walls. Calcium antagonists interfere with this entry of calcium into the cells. Hence, calcium antagonists relax the muscle in vessel walls and decrease resistance to blood flow and blood pressure. They act as a form of *vasodilator* (or "vessel dilator") as described in chapter 11.

However, calcium antagonists differ from other vasodilators in two important ways. First, they partially block signals from the nerves to the heart. This lessens the increase in heart rate that usually happens with vasodilators other than calcium antagonists. Second, calcium antagonists have a small diuretic effect (refer to chapter 7 for more on diuretics). The kidneys are less likely to retain fluid, a problem caused by other vasodilators. Therefore, calcium antagonists have some advantages over other vasodilators.

In fact, calcium antagonists have many ideal features for lowering blood pressure. Compared to some other blood pressure-lowering drugs such as diuretics, they don't have undesirable effects on blood lipids (cholesterol and triglycerides), blood potassium, sodium (salt), uric acid or glucose (blood sugar). More recent studies have shown that calcium antagonists also may have a beneficial, preventive effect on the development of atherosclerosis (hardening of the arteries caused by deposits of lipids and calcium inside the arteries).

Table 1 shows the three calcium antagonists currently available in Canada, both in regular and long-acting form.

Calcium antagonists can be separated into two classes. The drugs ending in "...dipine" (such as nifedipine) are more vasodilating and less heart-slowing, whereas others (verapamil and diltiazem) are more heart-slowing and have less vasodilating effect.

Table 1: Calcium Antagonists

Chemical name	Brand name	Average daily dose (mg)	Frequency of administration
Diltiazem	Cardizem	90–360	3/day
	Cardizem SR	90–360	2/day
Nifedipine	Adalat capsules	30–120	3–4/day
	Adalat PA tablets	20–120	2–3/day
Verapamil	Isoptin	240–480	2–3/day
	Isoptin SR	240–480	1–2/day

WHEN CALCIUM ANTAGONISTS ARE USED

In addition to their benefits for lowering blood pressure, calcium antagonists are useful for the treatment of angina. This is because they decrease the activity of the heart and therefore its work. Thus, for patients with both angina and high blood pressure, they may be a good choice. Calcium antagonists have been shown to be more effective in patients with low renin (for a brief description of the renin-angiotensin system, see chapters 1 or 9). This includes elderly and black people.

As nifedipine tends to accelerate the heart rate, its use with a beta-blocker is a good choice, provided the heart function is relatively normal (beta-blockers are described in chapter 8).

Calcium antagonists are also useful in lowering blood pressure when certain drugs (such as diuretics or beta-blockers) must be avoided because the patient has other medical conditions (e.g., asthma, high cholesterol/triglyceride levels, gout, Raynaud's disease, or diabetes).

WHEN CALCIUM ANTAGONISTS ARE AVOIDED

Currently available calcium antagonists may decrease the strength and frequency of heart contractions. If the heart is failing, these calcium antagonists can make this worse.

Verapamil and diltiazem should be used very carefully with beta-blockers. If they're combined with a beta-blocker, the electrical conduction in the heart may be slowed too much. Patients with prior problems with the electrical (impulse) conducting system of the heart should not be prescribed the currently available calcium antagonists, as their condition may worsen.

SIDE-EFFECTS OF CALCIUM ANTAGONISTS

Nifedipine, which acts a little like a vasodilator, can cause headaches, palpitations and flushing. These symptoms will usually decrease within a few weeks. The capsule form of nifedipine more often causes these side-effects, as the drug is rapidly absorbed and its quantity in the blood increases suddenly. In fact, the capsules can cause sudden large drops of blood pressure and dizziness. The tablets (Adalat PA) are absorbed slowly. The quantity of nifedipine in the blood then remains more constant and doesn't peak as much. In either case, use with a beta-blocker may prevent some of these side-effects.

Calcium antagonists, particularly nifedipine, may cause

ankle swelling. This is not due to water retention, as some of these drugs have a small diuretic effect on their own; rather, it's because of an effect on the small blood vessels. Therefore, adding a diuretic will not help.

Calcium antagonists may cause digestive disorders such as nausea, heartburn and infrequently, a decrease of appetite or diarrhea. Verapamil is particularly associated with constipation.

All these side-effects are reversible by discontinuing use of the drug.

11

Vasodilators

Louise F. Roy, M.D. and Frans H. H. Leenen, M.D., Ph.D.

HOW VASODILATORS WORK

This group of drugs relaxes the muscle of the blood vessel walls. The vessels dilate, and the resistance to the flow of blood within them decreases. (As you may recall from chapter 10, calcium antagonists act as vasodilators, but they also have other effects.)

If this dilation were the only effect, these drugs would be well suited for the treatment of high blood pressure. Unfortunately, they also have several other effects that fight their blood pressure-lowering action. They cause the kidneys to retain sodium (salt) and water, so the total water and sodium in the body increases. They also cause the heart to beat faster and more strongly. These last two consequences tend to partly overcome the beneficial effect of relaxing the blood vessels. They can also cause side-effects when these drugs are used alone.

In hypertension, the heart has to pump harder to overcome the higher resistance. Gradually it becomes larger. This increase in heart size (or *heart hypertrophy*) increases the risk of cardiovascular complications such as heart failure and sudden death. Fortunately, the heart size may return to normal if high blood pressure is being treated well. However, vasodilators used alone will let the heart work even harder, and heart size may not return to normal and may even get worse.

Two vasodilators, hydralazine and minoxidil, are available in Canada for the treatment of high blood pressure (see table 1). Other vasodilators are used only intravenously in the hospital.

Table 1: Common Vasodilators Used in Canada

Chemical name	Brand name	Average daily dose (mg)	Frequency of administration
Hydralazine	Apresoline	50–200	2-3/day
Minoxidil	Loniten	2.5–20	1-2/day

WHEN VASODILATORS ARE USED

Vasodilators usually aren't used alone; they're most often given with a beta-blocker and a diuretic. These combinations tend to overcome the side-effects of vasodilators on the kidneys and the heart, described above.

Hydralazine is one of the few drugs that can be used safely by pregnant hypertensive patients.

Minoxidil is a very potent drug to lower pressure. It's helpful when the blood pressure is very high and has been difficult to control with other drugs. Once the blood pressure settles down, other drugs are usually substituted, but sometimes it's necessary to continue with minoxidil.

WHEN VASODILATORS ARE AVOIDED

Vasodilators increase the work of the heart, making it beat faster and more powerfully. If you have angina, vasodilators may worsen it.

In recent years, we've seen the development of new classes of drugs that are easier to use and have fewer side effects. These drugs, such as calcium antagonists and ACE inhibitors, are replacing vasodilators.

SIDE-EFFECTS OF VASODILATORS

Headache, flushing and palpitations are frequent side-effects of vasodilators. These are sometimes temporary problems and disappear gradually by themselves or when the vasodilators are combined with beta-blockers. Vasodilators, when used alone, may worsen angina. Ankle swelling is another side-effect and is due to the retention of salt and water by the kidneys; a diuretic may counteract this.

In higher doses (300 mg or more per day), hydralazine may cause the patient to produce antibodies against his own body, resulting in painful, swollen joints. This is reversible, provided the drug was not used for too long.

Minoxidil may increase hair growth on the body. In fact, it's now made into an ointment and can be rubbed on the scalp to help with some forms of baldness. Bald people should use this ointment only if they have normal heart function, because some of the minoxidil is absorbed from the scalp and may increase the activity of the heart. In rare cases, water may accumulate in the envelope (*pericardium*) around the heart. These side-effects are reversible if minoxidil is stopped.

12

Hypertension in the Elderly

Pierre Larochelle, M.D., Ph.D. and A. Mark Clarfield, M.D.

High blood pressure is considered to be a major risk factor for the development of heart problems and diseases of the blood vessels in older people. There's no set definition of "older," although 65 is the starting age most often used. Studies that have looked at hypertension or other diseases have used various age groups, such as 65 - 74 years, 75 - 84 years, and 85 years and over, to help us understand the risks of high blood pressure and benefits of treatment in relation to age.

For the elderly, hypertension is defined as a blood pressure higher than 160 mmHg systolic and over 90 mmHg diastolic. At 160/90 mmHg, there's a small increase in risk of future cardiovascular disease. This doesn't necessarily mean that drug treatment has to be started at this level. However, the higher the pressure, the higher the risk, and the more likely that your doctor will start treatment.

The incidence of hypertension increases with age. Twenty-five percent of men and 30 percent of women over the age of 65 have a blood pressure higher than it should be. The systolic pressure (the higher pressure), in particular, increases with age. Although it was once thought that the diastolic pressure (the lower pressure) was more important, in older individuals the systolic pressure is a slightly better indicator of the level of risk. Thus, the systolic pressure is often given more weight in deciding when to treat an elderly hypertensive.

In some cases, the systolic pressure can increase without any change in the diastolic pressure (for example, 200/80 mmHg). This type of high blood pressure is called *isolated systolic hypertension.*

The blood pressure of anyone over 65 should be checked at least once a year. If it's higher than 160/90 mmHg, then more frequent readings should be taken by a nurse or a doctor to determine a proper course of action. Only if the blood pressure remains high for several readings may treatment be needed.

HYPERTENSION AND CARDIOVASCULAR RISK FACTORS

Several factors can lead to cardiac disease (heart failure, heart attack), stroke or an aneurysm (a weakening and swelling of the major blood vessel of the body, the aorta). In younger people, the biggest risk factors are cigarette smoking, high blood cholesterol and high blood pressure. In older people, high blood pressure is the most important risk factor for heart or vascular (blood vessel) disease.

EFFECTS OF HIGH BLOOD PRESSURE ON THE BODY

High blood pressure itself causes no complaints or symptoms in its early stages. However, if the high blood pressure is severe or remains untreated for a long time, damage to the heart, kidneys or brain may develop (as discussed in chapter 1).

Damage to the heart may cause shortness of breath, swelling of the feet, getting up more frequently during the night to pass urine, and sometimes pain in the chest (angina). Less often, these complaints can also occur in persons who have a normal blood pressure. When these symptoms are present, you must mention them to your doctor.

CAUSES OF HIGH BLOOD PRESSURE

Hypertension can be divided according to its causes. Most people (90 - 95 percent) with high blood pressure have essential hypertension; we don't really know what's causing it. It's likely that the hypertension is due to a combination of factors such as diet, environment and inherited abnormalities in the blood pressure regulating system. The other 5 - 10 percent of hypertensives have secondary hypertension, caused by diseases of the kidneys, the adrenal glands or of the blood vessels themselves (see chapters 1 and 2 for more details).

In those over age 65, additional factors come into play, the most important of which is a change in the structure of the major blood vessels. These become less elastic and more rigid, causing the systolic blood pressure to increase. This condition, known as *arteriosclerosis*, is the major cause of hypertension in this age group. Various other functions also change with age: blood vessels not only become more rigid but they also have difficulty relaxing and there's often a decline in the function of the kidneys.

With age, these factors can lead to a gradual increase in blood pressure. In many older people, however, no increase occurs, but if it does it should not be considered "normal," since it increases the incidence of heart problems and stroke.

INVESTIGATION AND DIAGNOSIS

The diagnosis of hypertension is discussed fully in chapter 2. The main difference for the elderly is the level of blood pressure used to make the diagnosis. A diagnosis of high blood pressure is made when the reading is above 160/90 mmHg on at least three different occasions, a minimum of one week apart. When the diagnosis is made, your doctor should make a detailed physical examination to determine the condition of your heart and blood vessels. Laboratory tests will include urine and blood samples to evaluate your kidney function and blood sugar level, as well as an electrocardiogram and possibly a chest X-ray.

BENEFITS OF TREATMENT

It has been proven that persons aged 65–80 who have hypertension and receive medications to lower blood pressure suffer fewer strokes and are less likely to have heart failure than those who don't receive medication. In fact, the studies indicate that this benefit is greater than in younger hypertensives. Nevertheless, drug treatment isn't without its own problems. The risks and benefits of treatment have to be weighed for each person. Patients with milder hypertension (systolic readings between 160 and 180 mmHg) may require only observation without treatment, unless the physical examination or blood tests reveal damage to the heart or blood vessels.

For those over 80, the benefits of treatment have not been so clearly established. Depending on your health and medications, your doctor may delay treatment to observe your condition before prescribing anything. He may even decide against treatment altogether.

We also don't know whether the treatment of isolated systolic hypertension is beneficial. A big study is currently in progress to answer this question. In the meantime, most doctors prescribe treatment for very high systolic pressures (above 200 mmHg).

Treatment, therefore, depends on your age, and, more importantly, on your health. Your medical history, symptoms, physical examination and laboratory tests will be considered along with the results of your blood pressure readings when you and your doctor decide on the treatment you should receive. For some people who experience adverse effects of medication, the potential benefits may not outweigh the harm, particularly if the blood pressure isn't greatly elevated.

TREATMENTS

Non-drug therapies

There have been no studies looking at the benefit of weight-loss in the treatment of high blood pressure in the elderly. Studies in the general population indicate that obesity is associated with an increased blood pressure and that, in younger patients, weight reduction can reduce blood pressure. However, because it's difficult for older people to lose weight, you are advised to follow a balanced diet and to at least ensure that you do not gain weight.

There are also no studies of the effectiveness of salt restriction in lowering blood pressure in the elderly. Nevertheless, you should reduce the salt in your diet as much as is practical, because high salt intake can interfere with the effectiveness of most medications in lowering blood pressure. An exception here is calcium antagonists: salt restriction may actually reduce their effectiveness.

Other forms of non-drug treatments have never been properly evaluated in older patients. However, consuming over 60 ml (2 oz) of alcohol per day (see chapter 5) is associated with increased blood pressure; thus, you should restrict alcohol use if your pressure is high. Exercise is also a general measure for well being. As much as possible, you should use walking or other forms of aerobic exercise to stay in shape, and they may be helpful in the control of blood pressure. If you wish to increase your exercise, your doctor can advise you and supervise your program.

Obviously, you should stop smoking, as continued smoking will cause further damage to your heart and blood vessels.

The importance of lowering cholesterol levels is not known in older individuals, although very high levels probably should be reduced when possible.

There is more complete information about non-drug treatments for hypertension in chapters 4 and 5.

Medications

Patients over the age of 65 who need drug treatment for their high blood pressure are prescribed the same types of medications as younger patients. A diuretic is usually the preferred medication to start treatment for hypertension in the elderly; however, the choice of treatment also depends on several other factors, as discussed in chapter 6.

To limit side-effects, the lowest possible dose will be prescribed. One of the main problems in treating hypertensive patients over 65 years of age is ensuring that the blood pressure is brought down as close as possible to normal levels without causing intolerable or dangerous side-effects. If you have an abnormal reaction to a medication, you should notify your doctor promptly so that a reduction or change in the medication can be considered. You should not stop taking the medication without advising your doctor because a sudden and dangerous rise in blood pressure could result.

CONCLUSION

Remember that a higher than normal blood pressure in an older person can contribute to cardiovascular disease. The risk increases as the level of the blood pressure increases and as the length of time that a person has had hypertension grows. Treatment can be useful to reduce the incidence of these complications. Nevertheless, the decision to treat and the choice of treatment must take into account your age, the level of your high blood pressure, your other medical problems and any medications that you're already taking.

13

Hypertension in Diabetics

Pavel Hamet, M.D., Ph.D. and Jean-Hugues Brossard, M.D.

WHAT IS DIABETES?

Diabetes is a disease in which the quantity of sugar (*glucose*) in the blood is elevated. Blood sugar is maintained at a stable level by the action of several hormones. One of these, insulin, is secreted by the pancreas. If the pancreas doesn't produce enough insulin, the blood sugar goes up (*Type 1 diabetes*). If the body produces insulin but the insulin doesn't work properly, the blood sugar also rises (*Type 2 diabetes*).

Type 1 (also called *insulin-dependent diabetes*) usually starts at a young age, in people below 30 years old. The survival of these patients depends on daily injections of insulin.

Type 2 (also called *non-insulin-dependent diabetes*) usually starts later in life, after 30 years of age. People with this problem still produce insulin, sometimes excessively. However, for various reasons including obesity, their insulin is less able to decrease blood sugar. Moreover, the quantity of insulin produced can also diminish with age. Although this form of diabetes can usually be treated by diet and medication, sometimes insulin injections are required.

TREATING DIABETES

Diabetes treatment begins with a special diet. For Type 2 diabetics, medication that lowers blood sugar (*oral hypoglycemic agents—hypoglycemia* means *low blood sugar*) may also be required. Insulin injections (one or more per day) are needed for allType 1 diabetics and for some people withType 2 diabetes.

There are two main goals of treatment. The first goal is the prevention of life-threatening high blood sugar. High levels of sugar in the blood can lead to coma (unconsciousness); before the discovery of insulin, this was often fatal for Type 1 diabetics.

The second goal is to keep blood sugar levels as normal as possible. Strict control of blood sugar prevents late complications, which can be a consequence of either Types 1 or 2 diabetes.

LATE COMPLICATIONS OF DIABETES

With time, diabetes affects blood vessels at two levels. When large arteries are affected, the complications are called *macrovascular.* When the small vessels (arterioles and capillaries) are affected, the complications are *microvascular.*

Macrovascular complications

Diseased large vessels progressively obstruct blood flow to the heart (coronary arteries), neck and legs. Symptoms vary, depending on the site of obstruction. They include angina and heart attack when the coronary arteries are affected, strokes when the neck arteries are obstructed, and cramps in the legs (claudication) on exercise when the leg arteries are narrowed.

Microvascular complications

Obstruction of small vessels (also known as *microangiopathy*) mainly affects the eyes and kidneys. The retina, at the back of the eye, is most affected by diabetes. Damage to the retina is called *retinopathy*. It's a serious complication of diabetes and causes 25 percent of all new cases of blindness.

Obstruction of small vessels in the kidney eventually causes kidney (renal) failure.

HYPERTENSION AND DIABETES

Quite frequently, diabetes is complicated by hypertension. Close to 50 percent of diabetics are hypertensive, and about 15 percent of hypertensive patients have problems with elevated blood sugar. The combination of hypertension and diabetes increases the chances of developing the complications described above. Furthermore, once complications are present, hypertension in diabetics increases the severity.

Although not many studies have been performed on the subject, it appears that diabetic hypertensive patients have more macrovascular complications, increasing the risk of angina, heart attack, stroke or poor circulation in the legs. This is true for both Type 1 and Type 2 diabetics. Hypertension also causes more rapid damage to renal function in Type 1 diabetics. Hypertension also increases the risk and severity of retinopathy in both types of diabetes.

TYPES OF HYPERTENSION IN DIABETES

Two types of hypertension can be distinguished in diabetes: essential hypertension, and hypertension associated with renal disease (*nephropathy*).

Essential hypertension that occurs in diabetics is probably of the same origin as in non-diabetics. Nevertheless, it has been demonstrated that diabetics have a greater tendency to retain salt. They also produce more adrenaline (which accelerates the pulse and blood pressure) in stressful situations, and they are also more susceptible to the effects of adrenaline. These three factors contribute to the development of hypertension in diabetics.

In nephropathy, the kidney doesn't function normally, and proteins are leaked from the blood into the urine. Hypertension in this situation is generally attributed to the renal disease. Thus, renal disease in diabetics leads to hypertension, and hypertension on its own can worsen the renal problem. This is a vicious circle with serious consequences.

BENEFITS OF CONTROLLING HYPERTENSION

There are many advantages in strictly controlling hypertension in diabetics. Several studies have demonstrated that hypertension therapy decreases protein losses in urine and slows the rate of kidney function deterioration. In this way, the vicious circle can be broken.

Good control of hypertension in diabetics decreases the risk of stroke. It may also slow the progression of retinopathy.

WHEN HYPERTENSION SHOULD BE TREATED

All diabetics with diastolic blood pressure exceeding 100 mmHg benefit from antihypertensive medication. If any vascular complications, including retinopathy and nephropathy, are detected, it's preferable to treat diastolic blood pressure of 90 mmHg or higher to slow their progression. Many doctors believe that all diabetics with diastolic pressure at or above 90 mmHg should be treated for high blood pressure even if there are no vascular complications.

WILL VASCULAR COMPLICATIONS APPEAR?

It has long been known that renal disease in diabetes starts with the leaking of certain proteins (albumin) from the blood stream into the urine in increasing quantities. Thereafter, renal function declines progressively. More recent studies have focused attention on the excretion of very small quantities of albumin (*microalbuminuria*). Microalbuminuria starts about 10 years before the development of major renal problems. It can also be a warning sign of retinopathy. With special lab tests, we can recognize at an early stage who is at risk of developing microvascular diabetic complications.

NON-DRUG TREATMENT FOR HYPERTENSIVE DIABETICS

Lifestyle changes

Having a healthy lifestyle (refer to chapter 5) and losing excess weight (refer to chapter 4) are essential. They help to decrease blood pressure and improve the control of blood sugar. Furthermore, the abnormal lipid (fatty substances in the blood) levels common in diabetes can frequently be improved. Decreased salt intake has added benefit because salt retention is a specific problem in diabetes.

Things to avoid

Certain medications should be avoided. Non-steroidal anti-inflammatory agents (such as ibuprofin, naprosin or in-domethacin) can have an adverse effect on renal function in diabetes. Corticosteroids (cortisone, prednisone) can lead to hypertension and decrease the control over blood sugar. Oral decongestants in cold remedies have effects similar to adrenaline, to which diabetics are particularly sensitive. All these medications can increase both blood pressure and blood sugar.

Consumption of alcoholic beverages can also elevate blood pressure. Furthermore, excessive alcohol intake can lead to serious hypoglycemia in diabetics treated with insulin.

DRUG TREATMENT FOR HYPERTENSIVE DIABETICS

As shown in table 1, several medications can be used to treat hypertension in diabetics. Most of them have specific advantages and disadvantages. We can classify them as "rather advantageous", "rather neutral" or "rather disadvantageous". Table 2 lists specific problems that diabetics face and the drugs that can make them worse.

Table 1: Drug Treatment of Hypertension in the Diabetic Patient

---

Medications for diabetics who do not take insulin,

in order of preference

- ACE inhibitors and/or calcium antagonists and/or beta-blockers with intrinsic sympathomimetic activity

- arterial vasodilators

- centrally acting agents

- loop diuretics with potassium-sparing properties

Medications usually to be avoided in Type 2 diabetes

- thiazide-like diuretics and beta-blockers without intrinsic sympathomimetic activity

- non-steroidal anti-inflammatory medications, corticosteroids, decongestants

---

Medications for diabetics treated with insulin,

in order of preference

- ACE inhibitors and/or calcium antagonists and/or thiazide-like diuretics

- alpha-blockers

- centrally acting agents

- loop diuretics and potassium-sparing diuretics

Medications to be avoided in Type 1 diabetes

- beta-blockers, particularly non-selective

Table 2: Conditions Aggravated by Antihypertensive Drugs

Condition	Drug
Control of blood sugar in Type 2 diabetes	diuretics beta-blockers
Suppression of symptoms of hypoglycemia	beta-blockers, mostly non-selective
Recovery from hypoglycemia	beta-blockers, mostly non-selective
Increase of lipids	diuretics beta-blockers without intrinsic sympathomimetic activity
Hyperkalemia	ACE inhibitors potassium-sparing diuretics
Impotence	Diuretics, beta-blockers (mostly non-selective), centrally acting agents
Orthostatic hypotension	centrally acting agents arterial vasodilators

Medications with advantageous effects

ACE inhibitors (captopril and enalapril). Several studies have shown that these medications (specifically captopril) decrease albumin in the urine of diabetics. Some of these studies have also demonstrated that captopril can slow the deterioration of renal function. ACE inhibitors don't elevate blood sugar or lipids, but they can increase blood potassium. Potassium tends to increase in some diabetics (a condition known as *hyperkalemia*), particularly older people with decreased renal and adrenal function. Generally speaking, ACE inhibitors are an excellent choice for the treatment of hypertensive diabetics.

***Calcium antagonists (diltiazem, nifedipine and verapamil)*.** Although these medications may slightly increase blood sugar when first taken, they don't do so with long-term use. They're also an excellent choice in the treatment of diabetics.

***Alpha-blockers (prazosin and terazosin)*.** These drugs don't affect blood sugar and, furthermore, they have advantageous effects on lipids. They can worsen the tendency of some diabetics to decreased blood pressure when standing (*orthostatic hypotension*). These medications are a good choice for most diabetics, although they have a limited hypotensive effect when used alone.

Medications with neutral effects.

***Arterial vasodilators (hydralazine and minoxidil)*.** Because they increase the heart rate and cause fluid to be retained in the body when used alone, these medications are usually given with a beta-blocker and a diuretic. They don't have any bad effects on blood sugar. They sometimes cause orthostatic hypotension.

***Potassium-sparing diuretics (amiloride, spironolactone and triamterene)*.** These medications can be given with other diuretics to avoid the loss of potassium. Given alone, however, they may cause increased levels of blood potassium in diabetics, particularly if there is any kidney impairment. They should not be given with ACE inhibitors, which can also cause potassium to rise.

Medications with disadvantageous effects.

Thiazide-type diuretics (hydrochlorothiazide, chlorothiazide, chlorthalidone and metolazone). These medications can increase blood sugar. They tend to make control more difficult in Type 2 (non-insulin-dependent) diabetics who are not taking insulin. This effect is in part due to *hypokalemia* (low potassium), which is frequently associated with their use. Hypokalemia leads to decreased insulin release by the pancreas and, consequently, to increased blood sugar levels. Furthermore, thiazides in high doses can elevate cholesterol and triglycerides (major blood lipids). They may also decrease sexual function, a frequent problem among diabetics. However, these medications, particularly in low doses, are still an acceptable choice in diabetics already treated with insulin.

Indapamide, another diuretic, may not have as severe adverse effects. It can be useful if a diuretic is needed for someone with Type 2 diabetes.

Loop diuretics (furosemide and ethacrinic acid). The role of these major diuretics is mainly to diminish salt and water retention in diabetics with renal failure. Outside this specific situation, their effects on blood pressure are not very potent.

Beta-blockers. Beta-blockers can cause several problems in diabetes. First, some of them increase lipids, particularly in diabetics not taking insulin (Type 2). This effect is probably absent with the use of beta-blockers that have intrinsic sympathomimetic activity (see chapter 8).

Second, beta-blockers (mostly non-selective) decrease the symptoms produced by hypoglycemia, which are due in great part to the effects of adrenaline. Diabetic patients with hypoglycemia will therefore have less increase in heart rate and few or no tremors or anxious feelings when using beta-blockers (particularly non-selective).

Third, beta-blockers (mostly non-selective) prolong the time needed by insulin-treated diabetics to recover from hypoglycemia.

Finally, adrenaline produced during hypoglycemia can lead to a severe increase of blood pressure if a person is taking a non-selective beta-blocker.

Clearly, for insulin-dependent diabetics prone to hypo-glycemia, non-selective beta-blockers can cause problems. For those not prone to hypoglycemia, beta-blockers can be very useful, especially those which are more selective such as atenolol, metoprolol and acebutolol.

Centrally acting agents (methyldopa and clonidine). These medications don't affect either blood sugar or lipids. However, they aggravate orthostatic hypotension and impotence in diabetics.

CONCLUSION

Diabetes and hypertension are common companions, and it's important to treat both well. Fortunately, there are very good treatments for hypertension that don't interfere with diabetes control; thus, it's usually possible to control both successfully.

14

Hypertension During Pregnancy or in Women who take Oral Contraceptives

Douglas R. Ryan, M.D. and Alexander G. Logan, M.D.

PREGNANCY AND HIGH BLOOD PRESSURE

High blood pressure occurs in about one percent of all pregnancies and can harm both fetus and mother. With early diagnosis and treatment, however, we can usually prevent problems.

Blood pressure normally falls during pregnancy due to a general relaxing of the mother's blood vessels. It reaches a low point about halfway through the pregnancy, and then slowly rises so that, at the mother's due date, her blood pressure has reached its non-pregnant level.

A woman is said to have high blood pressure in pregnancy if her blood pressure fails to show the usual mid-pregnancy fall, or if it's consistently higher than 140/90 mmHg.

Causes

Three conditions may produce high blood pressure during pregnancy: chronic hypertension, pre-eclampsia or gestational hypertension. The term *toxemia* is often used loosely to refer to any type of hypertension in pregnancy (most often pre-eclampsia). Since this term is not precisely defined, we recommend that it not be used.

Chronic hypertension.   This is high blood pressure that existed before pregnancy. Almost all women of childbearing age with this condition have essential hypertension, that is, high blood pressure without an identifiable cause. Women who are hypertensive before they become pregnant can remain hypertensive during their pregnancy. Sometimes their blood pressures may show a sharp rise in the last few months of the pregnancy. This poses a danger to mother and fetus alike.

Pre-eclampsia.   This condition arises only during pregnancy and disappears after the fetus is delivered. Pre-eclampsia is defined as the appearance of high blood pressure, ankle swelling, and protein in the urine during pregnancy. Pre-eclampsia occurs most often in the first pregnancy, and it seldom appears before the twenty-fifth week. It tends to run in families and occurs more often in mothers with chronic (long-standing) high blood pressure, chronic kidney disease, diabetes, multiple fetuses, or in mothers at the extremes of childbearing age (that is, teenagers or those over 35). Its exact cause is unknown, but it's associated with a general narrowing of the mother's blood vessels and a decrease in blood flow to the uterus (womb).

If the narrowing of blood vessels causes a decrease in blood flow to other body organs, then other symptoms and signs may occur. Headache, blurred vision, and eventual seizures may indicate brain involvement. Severe abdominal pain may be a sign of liver involvement. A decrease in urine production or a buildup in the blood of dietary waste products normally eliminated by the kidneys may show their involvement. Abnormal blood clotting may occur.

Although pre-eclampsia usually disappears quickly when the pregnancy ends, some of its features may persist. A small number of patients may show high blood pressure or protein in the urine for up to six months after delivery. If high blood pressure or protein in the urine persists beyond that time, they are probably not related to pregnancy. Additional investigation is required in this circumstance, especially if the mother was known to have normal blood pressure before conception.

Only one in ten mothers who have pre-eclampsia in their first pregnancy will develop it in a later pregnancy. Fewer than one in a hundred mothers who had a normal first pregnancy will develop pre-eclampsia in a subsequent one. The risk increases, however, if a subsequent pregnancy is conceived with a different father. Pre-eclampsia does not cause the development of high blood pressure later in life.

Gestational hypertension. This is defined as high blood pressure without ankle swelling or protein loss in the urine, occurring in a mother who had normal blood pressure before conception. It usually arises in the late stages of pregnancy and resolves within two weeks after delivery. It often recurs in later pregnancies. Unlike patients with pre-eclampsia, patients with gestational high blood pressure have a higher than average chance of developing high blood pressure later in life. It has been suggested that the tendency to hypertension in these women is temporarily unmasked by the stress of pregnancy.

Treatment

If high blood pressure is discovered during pregnancy, the doctor will first determine whether pre-eclampsia is present and, if so, its severity.

Chronic hypertension. If chronic high blood pressure becomes worse during pregnancy, the patient can usually be treated without having to go to hospital. Patients who are employed are usually advised to leave their jobs temporarily. All patients are asked to increase the amount of rest they're getting at home. Drugs that lower elevated pressures are then added as necessary.

Patients with chronic hypertension that remains poorly controlled (diastolic pressure greater than 100) are usually admitted to hospital for bed rest. Delivery is undertaken if the blood pressure is still not controlled or the fetus shows evidence of distress; delivery may also be undertaken if the fetus is mature. After delivery, higher doses of drugs may be required than before conception.

Treatment of chronic high blood pressure does not prevent the added development of pre-eclampsia, and your doctor will be constantly watching for this.

Pre-eclampsia. Women with pre-eclampsia are usually admitted to hospital for observation because this condition can change from mild to severe over 24–48 hours. Those with mild pre-eclampsia can be managed with bed rest and drugs that lower elevated pressures. Women with severe pre-eclampsia (severe blood pressure elevation and multiple organs involved) require treatment with intravenous medication and urgent delivery of the baby, as they will not improve until the pregnancy is ended. Left untreated, severe pre-eclampsia threatens the life of the mother and fetus.

Because many organs can be affected, pre-eclampsia in its early stages may be difficult to distinguish from chronic high blood pressure. Observation over time is often necessary to enable your doctor to decide.

Gestational hypertension. Women with gestational high blood pressure are treated in the same manner as those with pre-eclampsia (see above).

Drug therapy

Uncontrolled high blood pressure during pregnancy requires treatment. Antihypertensive therapy for all types of high blood pressure in pregnancy provides benefit to the mother and possibly the fetus. Most doctors prescribe medication when the mother's diastolic blood pressure is 100 mmHg or greater. The goal is usually a diastolic pressure of 80–90 mmHg; lower blood pressures may be potentially dangerous for the fetus as they may reduce blood flow to the uterus.

At least five different antihypertensive drugs have been well studied for use in pregnancy and are considered to be effective without endangering the development of the fetus. They are methyldopa, hydralazine, and three beta-blockers: oxprenolol, atenolol, and labetalol.

Therapy usually starts with one drug. A second and then a third drug are added if necessary. If the blood pressure can't be controlled with three drugs, it's unlikely to come down with the addition of more medication and delivery should be undertaken for the mother's safety.

Two types of drugs are usually avoided during pregnancy. Diuretics may increase the risk of low-birthweight infants. Angiotensin-converting-enzyme inhibitors, such as captopril and enalapril, may retard growth of the fetus. Other agents, including prazosin and calcium antagonists (such as nifedipine, diltiazem and verapamil) are not considered suitable because their safety has not yet been shown.

Recent reports suggest that pre-eclampsia may be prevented with a low dose of ASA given from 28 weeks gestation until delivery, but further study is needed before this can be recommended.

NURSING MOTHERS

Antihypertensive drugs taken after delivery by a mother who is breast-feeding are secreted into breast milk in tiny amounts. The daily dose received by a breast-feeding infant is about one hundredth that used to lower the mother's blood pressure. Not many scientific studies have examined the effects of breast-feeding and blood pressure medications. However, infants have routinely and successfully breast-fed from mothers taking methyldopa, hydralazine, oxprenolol, atenolol and labetalol. Diuretics are still avoided for treatment of high blood pressure after delivery as these drugs may decrease the amount of milk produced by the mother.

ORAL CONTRACEPTIVES

Oral contraceptives (birth control pills) are the most popular and effective form of temporary birth control. Because nothing else now available works as well, the pill will likely remain the most frequently used contraceptive for young women wishing to delay pregnancy. Oral contraceptives are also used in hormone replacement and to treat acne, excess body hair (*hirsutism*), menstrual irregularities (*dysmenorrhea*) and non-cancerous lumps in the breast. Oral contraceptives must be used with caution, however, because they sometimes cause important adverse effects, including blood pressure elevation.

Before prescribing oral contraceptives, your doctor will first enquire about your medical history and present health, and will discuss the risks and benefits of each method of contraception.

Oral contraceptives should not be prescribed to women with a history of *thrombophlebitis* (the formation of blood clots in the veins), stroke, heart attack, liver disease, known or suspected breast cancer, any estrogen-dependent tumor, abnormal uterine bleeding of unknown cause, or pregnancy or suspected pregnancy.

Blood pressure rises a little in virtually all women who take estrogen-containing oral contraceptives. This increase usually starts three to nine months after beginning the pill, and is not enough to matter for most women. Unfortunately, over a five-year period of pill use, the rise is enough to push the pressure beyond the 140/90 level in about five percent of women. In a very small number of women, the rise will be abrupt and will cause severe high blood pressure. The incidence of high blood pressure is lower when "mini-pills" containing lower doses of estrogen are used.

The way in which oral contraceptives cause high blood pressure is unknown. Most women gain weight when put on the pill, and salt and water retention in body tissue has been suggested as the cause of their increased blood pressure.

If your blood pressure rises by more than 10 – 20 mmHg while you are taking an oral contraceptive, it is usually advisable to stop taking the medication and to choose another method of birth control. Your blood pressure should return to normal within six months; if it doesn't, your doctor will make further tests for high blood pressure and may prescribe blood pressure lowering drugs. Such high blood pressure may not necessarily be caused by the oral contraceptives but may simply have developed about the same time.

High blood pressure is not an absolute reason to avoid using oral contraceptives, but other methods of contraception are preferable if you have hypertension. If you're unable to use another method, then medication to lower your blood pressure may be prescribed in addition to the oral contraceptive. This puts you in the awkward position, however, of taking one medication that raises your blood pressure and another that lowers it.

Oral contraceptives should not be prescribed for women over 35 years of age who smoke, because this combination leads to a high risk of cardiovascular disease. High blood pressure is a major part of this pill-associated risk. Another possible mechanism for the high risk is an increased tendency of the blood to clot. A third mechanism may involve changes in blood fats (lipids) caused by the pill.

The increase in risk depends on the type and dosage of the hormones in the oral contraceptive. Estrogens have a favorable effect on blood fats by raising the HDL-cholesterol ("good" cholesterol) and lowering LDL-cholesterol ("bad" cholesterol). Progestins, also contained in the pill, have the opposite effect.

Although hormones can cause or worsen high blood pressure in a small percentage of women over 55 years of age, in most cases they cause only a slight increase in blood pressure. This factor should nevertheless be taken into account in the case of patients taking estrogen to prevent or lessen menopausal symptoms or to prevent *osteoporosis* (thinning of the bones). The risks of hormone therapy are increased if the blood pressure is very high, or if the patient smokes or has a history of stroke.

In summary, you and your doctor should work together to avoid problems with the pill by observing the following precautions:

- Your doctor should prescribe the lowest effective dose of estrogen.

- Your doctor should give you no more than a six-month supply.

- You should have your blood pressure checked every six months and whenever you feel ill.

- If your blood pressure rises (above 140/90 mmHg, on average), you should stop the pill and use another form of contraceptive.

- If your blood pressure does not return to normal within six months of stopping the pill, you will need additional investigation and treatment.

15

How You Can Help Keep Your Blood Pressure Under Control

C. Edward Evans, M.B. and R. Brian Haynes, M.D.

With the treatments that we have today, no one need suffer the complications of high blood pressure. But many people do suffer from its effects because they don't follow the treatments prescribed by their doctor. This is tragic, because complications can be prevented by close teamwork between patient and doctor. This chapter will give you the information you need to keep up your end of the teamwork.

We'll begin with a short summary of our suggestions for self-help:

1. Take all your medication exactly as prescribed. To be sure that you do this:

    • Take your pills at the time of regular activities you do each day, such as brushing your teeth. We call this tailoring your treatment to fit your daily schedule.

    • Set out all your pills for the week on the first day of each week in a special pill organizer.

- If you miss *any* pills, be sure to let your doctor know on your next visit.

2. Refill your prescription *before* it runs out.

3. Make sure that you have a follow-up appointment with your doctor *before* you leave the office.

4. If you must miss an appointment, call your doctor's office to make another appointment as soon as possible.

5. Always keep an up-to-date list of your medication in your wallet.

6. Don't change the amount of your medication or how often you take it without first talking to your doctor. You can help with these adjustments by following these suggestions:

   - Let your doctor know about any side-effects.

   - Keep track of the times during the day or week when you tend to miss or forget your pills.

   - Measure your own blood pressure at home or have it taken at work.

7. Be sure to let your doctor know if you have any problems with or questions about the care you're receiving. Let your doctor know how you feel about your care and tell him if you're pleased with it.

MYTHS ABOUT HIGH BLOOD PRESSURE THAT CAN LEAD PEOPLE TO STOP TREATMENT

Before we discuss the reasons for these recommendations, we'd like to expose a few common myths about high blood pressure. If you already know what high blood pressure is and is not, you may want to skip this section on myths and go right to the action part of this chapter, entitled *WHAT YOU CAN DO TO KEEP YOUR BLOOD PRESSURE UNDER GOOD CONTROL.*

High blood pressure comes and goes

As stated earlier in this book, once it begins, high blood pressure is almost always a lifelong condition and will continue to cause problems if it's not treated. So, for the great majority of people with high blood pressure, it's necessary to continue treatment every day for the rest of their lives. We know from research studies that people who stop taking the treatment prescribed for them often do so because they don't know this important fact.

There are a few exceptions to the above rule. If your blood pressure is very well controlled on medication and stays well controlled for at least a year, your doctor may be able to reduce the amount of medication or even stop it for a period. If you feel that this may be your situation, it's a good idea to bring it to your doctor's attention. But it's important to know that your blood pressure should be checked even more often after any reduction in medication to make sure that it stays down. It's also important to remember that, although you may be able to get by on less medication, high blood pressure seldom goes away permanently.

Another way that high blood pressure can "disappear" is if its cause is removed. Unfortunately, as explained in chapters 1 and 2, finding a cause for a person's high blood pressure is rare.

High blood pressure can also be resolved the hard way: following a heart attack if the pumping power of the heart is damaged. You'll certainly know about this if it occurs; we hope it won't happen to you.

High blood pressure causes symptoms that tell you when you need to take your medication

Many people think that they can tell when their blood pressure is up from the way they feel. For example, they believe their blood pressure is up when they are feeling nervous, tense, or anxious, when they're red in the face, or when they have a headache or nosebleed. These are not good measures of your blood pressure! You can't feel anything going on in your blood vessels because they don't have the sort of nerve supply that produces feeling.

At the time that high blood pressure is discovered in most people, no symptoms have occurred, and very little or no permanent damage has been done. Usually the hypertension is detected during a routine blood pressure measurement, at a physical examination or when the pressure is checked during a visit to the doctor for some other reason. You can't use symptoms of tenseness — or any other feelings — to guide you in taking your prescribed treatment for hypertension. Believe it or not, what you feel is no help in letting you know whether your blood pressure is normal or high. Only a measurement of the blood pressure itself can tell you this, so you should not wait until you think your pressure is up to take medication. In addition, if you take your medication irregularly, you can cause your blood pressure to go on a "roller-coaster ride" that can, at times, be quite dangerous.

Your doctor can tell whether or not you are taking your medication

It's only natural that people try to keep the amount of medication they take for their high blood pressure (or any other medical condition, for that matter) as low as possible. This can often result in a somewhat dangerous game being played that goes as follows: first, the person cuts back his medication to, say, half the prescribed dose. Then, on the next visit to the doctor, the patient doesn't mention the reduced dose, hoping that the doctor will find that the blood pressure is well controlled anyway. If the blood pressure is elevated, the doctor then often thinks that the medication that he has prescribed isn't strong enough to do the job, and so the prescription is increased. The patient is now in a position where he either will have to confess to lowering the dose or will have to accept the new prescription and try to guess how much of it he should take to keep the blood pressure controlled.

This dangerous game can play out in another way: even though less medication has been taken, your blood pressure may be normal on the day of your visit to the doctor, and you and the doctor may think it's controlled. However, a single reading is not a good measure of your usual blood pressure. Multiple readings are needed to determine the usual blood pressure.

Research studies have shown that the most likely reason for poor lowering of blood pressure is that a person hasn't taken all the prescribed medication. Many doctors aren't aware that their patients have taken less than the prescribed amount of treatment. The only way your doctor can tell for sure how much medication you have missed is if you tell him. If you've missed any of your pills, for any reason, be sure to let your doctor know this when you visit.

Better still, you can help to keep the amount of medication prescribed to the smallest amount possible by taking all the medication that has been prescribed and bringing to the doctor a list of blood pressure readings taken between visits.

The side-effects of blood pressure medications are worse than the disease

All medications, by government regulation, have to be thoroughly tested before they can be prescribed. Drugs with serious side-effects (that is, side-effects that threaten your health) are generally weeded out by this procedure. Because high blood pressure is so common, doctors have a lot of experience with blood pressure drugs and can avoid ones with important or common side-effects. As a result, only about one in five people experience any side-effects from the medications and most of these are usually just a nuisance rather than a danger. Side-effects almost always disappear once the drug is stopped and, because there are many drugs for hypertension, the medication can be changed easily if important or even merely annoying side-effects occur.

Nevertheless, like many people, you may feel a bit worse after you start blood pressure medication. This could be partly because you now know that you have a chronic disease and begin to blame it for many of the aches and pains of everyday existence. It also may take some time for your system to adjust to the medication. You may experience some light-headedness upon standing, or a bit of drowsiness or lack of energy after starting some blood pressure lowering pills. But these reactions will usually pass with time as your body becomes used to the lower blood pressure and the new medication.

Most people whose blood pressure is well controlled on medication continue their normal lifestyle without any restrictions. On the other hand, some people do experience side-effects from medication and need a change in dose or drug.

The only way that your doctor can know whether your reactions mean that your medication needs to be changed is if you let him know exactly what you have experienced. You can help your doctor find the best treatment for you by keeping track of any important symptoms that you feel may be due to your medication. Write them down between visits so you will be able to describe them clearly when you meet with your doctor.

Many people don't want to bother the doctor by complaining about side-effects. This concern about hurting the doctor's feelings or wasting his time is very considerate but not very wise. We know that patients who like their doctors are less likely to let them know about important complaints than those who aren't so devoted to their doctors. Would you fail to notify the garage if the headlights weren't working after your car had been serviced? Of course not! So be sure to have your side-effects attended to, if and when they occur.

One last word: if you do experience side-effects that are not severe, don't stop or change your medication without talking to your doctor first. It goes without saying that if you experience severe side-effects, you should contact your doctor immediately.

High blood pressure is usually due to stress and/or bad diet; improving your lifestyle is better treatment than medication

While acute stress can raise your blood pressure for a short time, there's no evidence that stress can produce long-lasting high blood pressure. There are several non-drug treatments that people use to try to get their blood pressure down; they've been discussed in previous chapters, especially chapters 4 and 5. They include losing weight, reducing the amount of salt in the diet, lowering alcohol intake, and a variety of stress management techniques including relaxation, exercise, yoga, meditation, and biofeedback.

Most people find that attempting to make lifestyle changes is a lot more difficult than taking medication. Your doctor may prescribe one or more of these methods as a way to lower the amount of medication that you have to take. If this is the case, do your best to follow the recommendation, but it's very important that you realize that non-drug treatments are often no substitute for drug treatments if your blood pressure is more than mildly elevated.

Your doctor won't be satisfied with your treatment until your blood pressure is well controlled — and neither should you. If your doctor starts you on a non-drug treatment without also putting you on medication, be sure to attend all follow-up visits. If your blood pressure doesn't fall to normal levels in a few weeks, go along with your doctor's suggestion to go on medication. This is not a failure on your part; it doesn't mean that your high blood pressure is unusual; and it isn't necessary to give up the improvements you have been able to make in your lifestyle.

If you have high blood pressure, you must "take it easy" and avoid stress or exertion.

No way! If your blood pressure is controlled by medication, then you can lead a perfectly normal existence. You need take no more time off work because of stress or colds than if you did not have high blood pressure. You can practise whatever recreation you like except weight lifting.

Remember, hypertension is a completely symptomless and painless disorder. If it's caught early in its course, it stays that way as long as it's kept under control.

WHAT YOU CAN DO TO KEEP YOUR BLOOD PRESSURE UNDER GOOD CONTROL

On the surface, keeping your blood pressure under control appears to be a simple enough job: keep all your appointments and take your treatments as they have been prescribed by your doctor. However, because you must carry out these tasks for the rest of your life, this may be a lot more difficult than you imagine. In fact, without special help, only one person in five does a really good job of following the prescribed treatment for such a long period. The following steps will help you with the lifelong job of keeping your blood pressure under control:

- Clear up any doubts you may have about following the treatment.

- Use special pill containers.

- Tailor your pill-taking so it fits your usual daily activities.

- Avoid running out of pills.

- Keep an up-to-date list of your medications with you at all times.

- Never leave the doctor's office without setting your next appointment.

- Keep track of your blood pressure.

- Measure your own blood pressure.

- Build a good working relationship with your doctor.

Clear up any doubts you may have about following the treatment

An individual is not likely to follow his prescription very closely if he has any doubts about whether or not he really needs to follow the treatment. It's very important to develop a strongly positive attitude that you are going to get the most out of the treatments your doctor prescribes. Hypertension has serious consequences if it isn't controlled, and you are at definite risk of its complications as long as your blood pressure remains high. The treatments for it are effective if they're taken as prescribed. Taking them is a nuisance, can be expensive, and is not without risks, but for most people, the benefits of treatment far outweigh any disadvantages.

Use special pill containers

Many people find it difficult to remember at 10:00 a.m. whether they took the dose of medication that they usually take at 8:00 a.m. One way to overcome this common problem is to buy a pill container with separate compartments for each day of the week. There are many such devices available from your pharmacist. On the first day of each week, fill each compartment of this container with all the pills that you'll need for the week. Then, if you can't recall later in the day whether you took your morning pill, just look in the compartment for the appropriate day and see whether the pill is present or "missing in action."

Another way is to buy a small pill container that will fit easily into your pocket or purse. Fill it up each morning with your pills for the day. Then if you can't remember whether you took your noon pills, just open the container and peek inside.

If you find that you're missing pills more than once a week, try to identify a pattern. Is it the pills you're supposed to take while at work that you're likely to miss? What about the pills you should take last thing at night? Or are weekends the most difficult? This way you may notice a particular time that you're more likely to miss taking your pills. If so, try the following suggestions.

Tailor your pill-taking so it fits your usual daily activities

Connect your pill-taking to regular events in your daily schedule so you take your pills at the same time every day. Do you have any daily habits — something you do every day of the week, whether you go to work or not — such as brushing your teeth every morning? Do you always have a cup of coffee or juice when you get up? Whatever your daily routine might be, link your pill-taking to that event. And, if you must take your pills more than once a day, think of a habit that coincides with those times and take your medicine then. A typical schedule might look something like this:

- breakfast: pill(s) and juice *before* the meal.
- supper: pill(s) and water or milk *before* the meal.
- bedtime: pill(s) and water *before* brushing your teeth.

Many people believe that different types of medications need to be taken at completely separate times. In fact, this is seldom so. For example, suppose you are prescribed three different medicines for your high blood pressure, all of which are to be taken once a day. You can (and should) take all of these pills at the same time unless your doctor or pharmacist advises otherwise. Another good idea is to try to schedule taking your pills when you're more likely to be at home. It's much harder to remember to take pills when away from home because of preoccupation with other activities or embarrassment about taking pills in public places.

If you do have to take your pills while at work, one suggestion already mentioned is to buy from your pharmacist a small pill container that you can keep in your pocket. Another is to keep a small extra supply of pills in your car or at work so you'll always have some on hand if you forget to bring some from home that day.

If you happen to miss a dose and you recall having missed it within a few hours, take it right away unless the next dose is scheduled to follow in a short while. For example, if you realize at suppertime that you missed your morning pill, and your next pill is not due until bedtime or the next morning, immediately take the pill that you missed.

Never run out of pills

Avoid running out of pills. Sometimes it happens that your doctor doesn't prescribe enough to last you until the next appointment, or you may have to postpone an appointment and your pills run out before the rescheduled time.

You may even feel that it won't make much difference if you stop the pills for a few days — after all, shouldn't your body take a rest from the pills occasionally? While this may sound logical, it's not correct and is potentially dangerous. In the first place, your body needs the pills to keep your blood pressure under control. Second, in some instances, stopping the medication suddenly can lead to sharp, severe rises in blood pressure that can be harmful. It isn't wise to stop your medication without your doctor's recommendation and careful measurement of your blood pressure. Therefore, if you ever find yourself without enough pills to last until your next appointment, make sure to have your prescription refilled before it runs out.

Here are some ways to avoid running out:

- When you visit your doctor, don't leave without a prescription for enough medication to last you until your next scheduled visit.

- When you're about to go on a vacation or trip, remember to take along all the medication you'll need, with a good margin for an unexpected delay. Make sure that you pack your pills someplace where you can easily get them at the right time.

- If you're about to run out of pills, either call your doctor's office directly, leaving the exact details of your prescription plus the phone number of the pharmacy, or call your pharmacist and ask him to call your doctor for a renewal. In either case, it's wise to allow two or three days for the prescription to be renewed.   But, if you do happen to run out before you notice it and you can't reach your doctor, your pharmacist will often provide you with enough pills to last you until the doctor can be contacted.

This is one situation in which an ounce of prevention is truly worth a pound of cure. It makes good sense to renew your prescription well before you run out and to avoid the hassle of having to scramble around at the last minute.

Keep an up-to-date list of your medications with you at all times

It's a good idea to keep an up-to-date record of your medications in your wallet or purse. There are several good reasons for this. Knowing something about the medications that you take can help make you feel more in control. If you're in an accident or become ill and require emergency medical aid, this information could be of vital importance in your care.

Should you lose or misplace your medication, especially if you're away from home, having a list handy can turn a possible disaster into a minor inconvenience. If you change doctors for any reason or are referred to another doctor for care of any problem, including your high blood pressure, your new doctor will want to know exactly what medications you have been prescribed. You can also use your list to check the accuracy of the prescription label when your medications are renewed. Doctors and pharmacists are human and sometimes make mistakes. They would prefer to have them pointed out before they cause you any grief.

To make it easier to follow this advice, ask your doctor or pharmacist to write down your medications on a piece of paper or a card. Or write them down yourself by copying them from the pill bottles you're given by the pharmacist. If you do this, ask your doctor or pharmacist to check your list. Of course, you should revise this list every time the medications are changed.

Never leave the doctor's office without setting up your next appointment

It's very important never to leave your doctor's office without a specific appointment for your next visit, and, if at all possible, never miss an appointment. It's very easy to drop out of care, and this is the most common cause of people failing to get and keep their blood pressure under control. If you don't have a specific appointment time and date when you leave your doctor's office, there's a good chance that you'll forget to make a new appointment for the appropriate time later. Sometimes you won't know what your schedule is going to be far enough in advance to make a definite appointment. If this is the case, it's worthwhile to make an appointment anyway when you think you might be able to attend. Then, if necessary, you can always phone back and change the appointment time.

With the active and busy lives most of us lead, remembering appointments can be a real problem. This is even more difficult if the date is several weeks or months in advance. If your doctor's office doesn't have an automatic reminder system (and most don't) then try developing one yourself. Each time you visit your doctor, be sure to write down the details of your next appointment before you leave. Even if the receptionist offers you the "opportunity" of calling back later for the next appointment, ask for a specific date and time if at all possible. If this isn't possible, write a reminder to yourself in your calendar or post it on the refrigerator. It's better to list the month and day, not "in two months' time," as you can easily forget which two months. When you get closer to the appointed time, then you can call to confirm it.

By the way, if you do miss an appointment, it's unlikely that the doctor's office staff will contact you. Most doctors consider it your responsibility to re-book missed appointments.

Keep track of your blood pressure

Many people find it helpful to see how well they're keeping their blood pressure under control. This provides feedback that can help to motivate your efforts to follow the treatment prescribed and may help with adjustments of your treatment.

Aside from the blood pressures taken when you visit your doctor's office, you can get more readings taken at work if you're employed somewhere with a nurse or other medical staff on duty. Many doctors also will allow (and encourage) you to drop into the clinic for a quick blood pressure check by the clinic nurse. Keep a record of all these blood pressures and show them to your doctor at your next visit. Aside from the picture they give you of your blood pressure control, they can provide your doctor with valuable information for adjusting your medications. This is because blood pressure varies a great deal from time to time, and readings taken outside the doctor's office are often a more accurate reflection of true blood pressure. The larger the number of blood pressure readings available to your doctor when decisions are made, the easier it will be to decide.

Measure your own blood pressure

For many people with hypertension, there are good reasons to invest in equipment to take your own blood pressure at home. The Canadian Coalition for High Blood Pressure Prevention and Control recommends self-measurement of blood pressure, under the guidance of a healthcare provider, in the following patients:

- Those who show labile (changing) or elevated blood pressure in the healthcare provider's office.

- Those with poorly controlled hypertension.

- Those who wish to play a greater role in their own care.

- Those who require an assessment of their antihypertensive therapy (blood pressure medication) because of concerns about excessive blood pressure lowering or insufficient duration of drug action.

Some people have high blood pressure time and again in the doctor's office, but when their blood pressure is measured away from the clinic, at home or at work, it's normal. We now know this "white coat" or "office" hypertension may not be as harmful as blood pressure that is high all the time. Home blood pressure measurement can be helpful in sorting out whether you have this type of high blood pressure.

If your doctor has suggested you take your pressure at home, or you would like to do it for your own interest, the first question usually is: which blood pressure machine should I get and where should I get it? Good question! One type of instrument has a column of mercury and is known technically as a *mercury sphygmomanometer* (see figure 1). Most people will recognize this as the type most commonly used by health professionals. The next most common type is the *aneroid sphygmomanometer*, which usually has a small round dial instead of a mercury column (see figure 2). You need a stethoscope to use either of these machines.

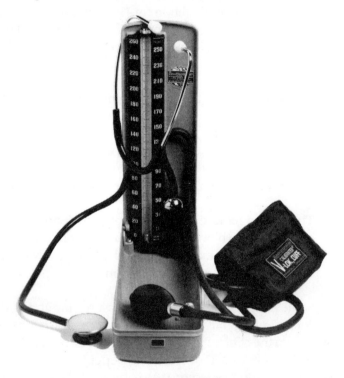

Figure 1: Mercury sphygmomanometer.

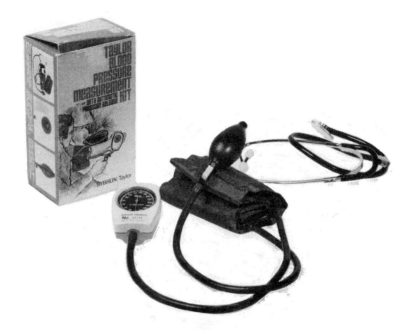

Figure 2: Aneroid sphygmomanometer.

Then there is a host of machines sold specially for home measurement. Many have digital displays. Most don't require the use of a stethoscope. Some automatically blow up the cuff and even deflate it. Some print out the pulse rate, systolic and diastolic blood pressures, date and time, and even have a built-in alarm clock!

Because many of these instruments are not reliable, we'd like to give you some guidance on which devices to buy and point you to sources of further information.

The most reliable and accurate type of machine, when it's used properly, is the mercury sphygmomanometer. This type is used as the standard against which other devices are measured. Baumanometer is a reputable maker of mercury devices, and you can buy their home blood pressure kit from surgical supply houses for about $100. The main drawbacks with mercury devices are that they are cumbersome and quite heavy, the mercury can spill out if the device is turned upside down or broken, and mercury can be very toxic. Added to this is the fact that you need to use a stethoscope, place it correctly on the arm, and listen for the sounds in the artery while reading the gauge and simultaneously deflating a cuff wrapped around one of your arms. Nevertheless, if you want to do the job properly, this is the way to go.

A good quality aneroid device is probably the next most commonly recommended. The advantage of an aneroid instrument over a mercury one is that it's much smaller and easier to handle and doesn't have the potential problem of mercury toxicity. It still requires the use of a stethoscope and juggling with deflation valves while reading the circular gauge. The other problem is that dropping it or rough usage can cause it to become inaccurate, and the only way of checking it is to take it back to your supplier or doctor and have it calibrated against (yes, you guessed it) a mercury sphygmomanometer.

With both of these machines, you need practice at measuring blood pressure the correct way. Table 1 outlines the approved method of taking blood pressure using a mercury or aneroid device, but you will most likely need someone who is familiar with taking blood pressure to show you how to do it. Don't give up if you find it difficult at first; most doctors and nurses couldn't hear a thing either when they were first taught to take blood pressures!

What about all the other fancy machines you see for sale (such as the one in figure 3) in department store catalogues, drugstores, electronics stores, and even advertised with your gas credit card bill? They certainly look attractive, hi-tech and simple to use, and usually don't need a stethoscope. If they are as accurate as the digital readout display leads you to believe, they could be the no-fuss answer, especially for people with a hearing impairment. Buyer beware! Many of these machines are so inaccurate that they can be positively dangerous. But there are so many potential advantages to an easy-to-use automatic machine that we can't dismiss them out of hand.

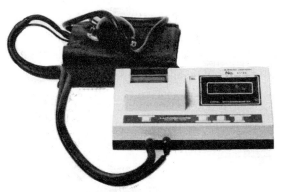

Figure 3: Digital home blood pressure device.

If you're thinking of buying your own blood pressure monitor, there are several articles that you can consult. (Information is given in the bibliography at the end of this chapter.) The Consumers' Association of Canada (CAC) published a review of electronic blood pressure monitors in the February 1987 issue of *Canadian Consumer.* In May 1987, the Consumers' Union of the United States published a similar review in their magazine *Consumer Reports.* Both of these articles should be available in your local public library and are well worth reading before you take the plunge.

A more detailed study of home blood pressure devices, but one that may be a little more difficult to get hold of, is a paper we published in the *Journal of Hypertension* in February 1989. We tested 23 different devices; the retail cost of the recommended machines was as low as $40 and as high as almost $300. Some recommended makes include Almedic, Astropulse, Lumiscope, Radio Shack, Sunbeam and Tyco.

Other points worth noting:

- Machines using microphones as the listening device have to be more carefully positioned on the arm than those using an oscillometer (a second bladder inside the cuff).

- Any machine for self-measurement of blood pressure should have a cuff that's specially made to be applied with one hand. Most use a bar called a D-ring and Velcro fasteners to make application easier.

- Electronic machines can give erratic readings when the batteries are getting low, and this usually happens *before* the battery indicator lets you know that the batteries need changing.

- Even though a good set of instructions may come with the machine, it's very important to review how to use it with someone who is well versed in taking blood pressures, such as your doctor or nurse.

- It's important to make sure you have the correct cuff size for your arm (see table 1).

- Most electronic instruments are very delicate, and if you drop one you should have its accuracy checked.

- Automatic blood pressure machines have real difficulty getting accurate readings if you have an irregular pulse or if your pulse is very slow.

- If you buy any blood pressure machine, insist on the right to return it if you're unable to get good readings at home or if it appears to be inaccurate when tested against your doctor's blood pressure machine.

Table 1: How to Measure Blood Pressure

1. If you are using a mercury sphygmomanometer, the top of the column should be at eye level.

2. Use a cuff that is the right size around the mid upper arm:

Adult arm size	Bladder size
less than 33 cm (13 in)	12x23 cm (5x9 in)
33–41 cm (13–16 in)	15x33 cm (6x13 in)
more than 41 cm (16 in)	18x36 cm (7x14 in)

3. Place the cuff with the lower edge 3 cm above the crease of your elbow with the bladder centred just inside your biceps muscle. You should be comfortable, with your arm bared and well supported.

4. Place the head of the stethoscope gently but firmly over the inside of your biceps muscle, just below the cuff. (If you squeeze this area with your fingers, you should be able to feel the brachial artery just to the body side of your biceps muscle, just above the crease of your elbow.)

5. Raise the pressure in the cuff about 30 mmHg above your usual systolic pressure.

6. Open the valve to let the air out slowly, about 2 mm per second.

7. Record the systolic pressure (2 mm above the first appearance of a clear tapping sound) and the diastolic pressure (2 mm above the point at which tapping sound disappears).

8. Ignore any isolated extra heartbeats or noises other than the regular tapping heart sounds.

9. Leaving the cuff partially inflated for too long may make the sounds disappear due to venous congestion. To avoid this, at least 30 seconds should elapse between readings. If the sounds are faint, raise your arm, milk down the forearm (i.e., encircle it with your fingers and firmly stroke down), and, with your arm still raised, inflate the cuff. Lower your arm and proceed to take your pressure.

10. If there is consistently higher pressure in one arm than the other, use the arm with the higher pressure.

If you do collect blood pressure readings between visits to your doctor, be sure to record the date and time of day, and show the results to your doctor. You can write down the pressure in a pocket calendar, along with any pills you may have missed and any side-effects you feel may have been due to the medication. This will make it possible to cover all these matters quickly with your doctor.

Blood pressure varies quite a bit from day to day and even from one hour to the next. For example, your blood pressure may be 140/96 on one reading and 120/80 the next. It's quite usual for the lower number of each of these two readings (i.e., 96 and 80, the diastolic blood pressures) to vary within a range of 20 — say, from 80 to 100 or 70 to 90. Because of this change from one time to the next, blood pressure is always taken as the average of several readings over a period of days or weeks. This is one of the reasons why it can be valuable for your doctor to have you record blood pressures between office visits. If these readings are accurate, they will provide more information on which to judge your average blood pressure.

It's very important for you to know that this variability in blood pressure exists so you don't become concerned about it or react incorrectly to it. Don't try to change your medication on the basis of the readings that you get, and don't be surprised if your blood pressure is up when you feel well or down when you feel tense. Rely on your doctor to interpret your blood pressures and you can be sure your readings will help make his job easier.

If you're monitoring your own blood pressure, you should discuss with your doctor how low a pressure you should aim for. For most people, the goal is to keep the average diastolic blood pressure below 90.

Build an effective working relationship with your doctor

Since you can expect that you'll require lifelong care for your hypertension, it's very important to establish a good relationship with your doctor. As with all relationships, this will require mutual effort if it is to be fully successful.

Most patients look for a doctor they can talk to who is interested in listening to their concerns. You should not be afraid to ask questions about your condition. Some doctors may be taken aback at first and even feel that they're being put on the spot, but most doctors will respond positively when they realize that you have genuine questions and concerns. For example, if you've been following a prescribed treatment faithfully and your blood pressure remains persistently elevated, it's perfectly all right to ask your doctor whether there is something more that can be done.

It's important to be honest and open with your doctor and to build a working relationship that will allow you to achieve all the benefits of modern therapy. This could be the beginning of a long and rewarding association. As in all relationships, if you're pleased with the care you're receiving, let your doctor know — you'll make his day. But, if you find you can't relate to your doctor and aren't getting the interest in or answers to your questions, get another doctor. After all, everyone has a different personality, and sometimes it takes a while to get a good match.

BIBLIOGRAPHY

"Blood pressure monitors." *Consumer Reports* (May 1987): 314-319.

Canadian Coalition for High Blood Pressure Prevention and Control. "Recommendations on self-measurement of blood pressure." *Canadian Medical Association Journal,* Vol. 138, No. 12 (15 June 1988):1093-6.

"Electronic blood pressure monitors." *Canadian Consumer* (February 1987): 21-24.

Evans, C. E., R. B. Haynes, C. H. Goldsmith, and S. A. Hewson. "Home blood pressure measuring devices: a comparative study of accuracy." *Journal of Hypertension,* No. 7 (1989):133-142.

Index

Yes!

I want to support The Canadian Hypertension Society (CHS) and their programs for research, treatment and education. (The CHS, established in 1979, is a non-profit organization.) Your support is appreciated and a tax receipt will be sent to you.

Enclosed is my cheque or money order payable to THE CANADIAN HYPERTENSION SOCIETY for:

☐ $10   ☐ $20   ☐ $50   ☐ $100   ☐ Other $____

Would you like to receive free copies of the quarterly newsletter of the CHS, Hypertension Canada?

☐ Yes   ☐ No

My name and mailing address are as follows:

Name _____

Address _____

_____

Send to:

Dr. E. Schiffrin
Secretary Treasurer
Canadian Hypertension Society
Clinicial Research Institute of Montréal
110 avenue des Pins, ouest
Montréal, Québec
H2W 1R7